# Health Care Systems of the Developed World

# Health Care Systems of the Developed World

*How the United States' System
Remains an Outlier*

DUANE A. MATCHA

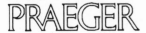

Westport, Connecticut
London

362.10973
M42h

**Library of Congress Cataloging-in-Publication Data**

Matcha, Duane A.
   Health care systems of the developed world : how the United States' system
remains an outlier / Duane A. Matcha.
      p.   cm.
   Includes bibliographical references and index.
   ISBN 0–275–97992–X
   1. World health. 2. Medical care—United States. 3. Medical care—Cross-
cultural studies. 4. Medicine—Cross-cultural studies. I. Title.
RA441.M38      2003
362.1′0973—dc21        2002193116

British Library Cataloguing in Publication Data is available.

Library of Congress Catalog Card Number: 2002193116
ISBN: 0–275–97992–X

First published in 2003

Praeger Publishers, 88 Post Road West, Westport, CT 06881
An imprint of Greenwood Publishing Group, Inc.
www.praeger.com

Printed in the United States of America

∞™

The paper used in this book complies with the
Permanent Paper Standard issued by the National
Information Standards Organization (Z39.48–1984).

10 9 8 7 6 5 4 3 2 1

# Contents

# Illustrations

## FIGURES

# Preface

The origin of this book lies in the construction some years ago of a new course I developed entitled Comparative Health Care Systems. As the title implies, the course examines selected health care systems located within the developed world, Eastern Europe, and the developing world. The course is a macro-level analysis of the structure and delivery of health care services as well as the implications associated with each system relative to the populations they serve.

Although health system analysis is an increasingly popular academic and nonacademic area of study, the application of a sociological interpretation is too often missing from the available data. Nevertheless, this is a particularly fascinating area of investigation. For example, consider the ongoing debate regarding the American health care system. Although the core issue is that of health, students are exposed to those social, political, and economic interests associated with the current health care system as well as the ramifications associated with its alteration. For instance, even though the American economy has experienced an unprecedented period of growth, the growing number of uninsured represents an ongoing problem. The uninsured, however, are not a homogeneous subpopulation, but rather represent a diverse coalition of young people, the working class, and a growing number of middle-class individuals and families unable to afford the increasing monthly health insurance premium. The growing economic differentiation among population groups will exacerbate already known health outcomes based on social class position. Thus, by framing the variables and their consequent analysis, it is possible to provide the reader with a sociological explanation of a highly complex and multidisciplinary area of study.

Although I try to remain as objective as possible relative to the benefits and limitations associated with each system, I am particularly critical of the American health care system. I consider the American health care system woefully inadequate and currently incapable of ensuring the health needs of the general population. Unfortunately, given contemporary American history and the current reality of a politically conservative Congress and president, there is little reason to believe significant change of the current system will occur. Instead, any alteration of the American health care system will occur incrementally. Although such an approach may pacify those with a vested interest in maintaining the status quo, those most impacted by the inefficiency and ineffectiveness of the health care system are becoming increasingly outspoken but politically invisible.

The book is more than a critique of the American health care system. It offers the reader insight into the differences among a select number of health care systems and an examination of outcomes associated with each system relative to a common core of sociological variables (age, sex, social class, and race and ethnicity). It is my belief that such an approach better serves the needs of students at all levels as they experience, generally for the first time, the dynamic qualities associated with health system analysis. The selected countries (exclusive of the United States) employ either a Bismarck (social insurance) or a Beveridge (national health insurance) health care system model. I am focusing on these models because they represent the primary types of health care systems currently in existence within the industrialized world.

In the final chapter I address the future of health care systems within the developed world. For some time the general consensus has been that health care systems will converge into an integrated model that incorporates features of existing systems. Although some evidence suggests such a movement is underway, there is an increasing literature base indicating system modification rather than convergence. What we do know, however, is that system-level changes are less the result of an integrative belief regarding the well-being of citizens and more the use of political pressure to reduce governmental involvement in health care.

This book is designed for a number of uses. It may function as a supplement to my *Medical Sociology* text (particularly chapter 13) or any standard text in medical sociology. This book may also be used as one in a series of books for any course that engages in health care system analysis. The length of the book was intentionally limited to approximately two hundred pages to allow greater flexibility and adaptation depending on the needs of individual faculty. Given the number of pages available, the choice was to attempt a cursory evaluation of health care systems across a large number of countries or provide a solid sociological foundation of those health care systems currently employed within the most economically advanced nations. I preferred the latter.

# Acknowledgments

As always, there are a number of people to thank. Siena College has continued to support my efforts to balance teaching responsibilities and scholarly endeavors by providing course-load reductions for all of my books. Jane Garry, Greenwood Publishing Group senior editor, and her assistant, Melissa Festa, deserve considerable praise for their efforts to bring this work to fruition.

Any shortcomings of this book lie with the author. As with previous books, I encourage responses from all readers. My e-mail address is matcha@siena.edu. Enjoy.

# CHAPTER 1

# Introduction

Every country has a national health system, which reflects its history, its economic development, and its dominant political ideology.

(Roemer 1993: 335)

## INTRODUCTION

The twenty-first century will challenge the ingenuity and integrity of health care systems throughout the industrialized world. Although any number of factors can be identified as the reason for this challenge, one of the most important lies in the fundamental shift in the economies of the industrialized world from industrial to computer-based technologies. Although this shift has been underway for some time, it is increasingly creating the foundation for significant economic opportunities as well as dislocation.

This economic transformation is also the impetus for an alteration of the sociopolitical environments toward what is referred to as postmodernism. This paradigmatic shift, evident in the broad-based social changes occurring throughout the industrialized world, is illustrated by the following statement:

[T]he Postmodern shift is a move away from both traditional authority and state authority. It reflects a declining emphasis on authority in general—regardless of whether it is legitimated by societal or state formulae. This leads to declining confidence in hierarchical institutions. Today, political leaders throughout the industrialized world are experiencing some of the lowest levels of support ever

recorded. This is not simply because they are less competent than previous leaders. It reflects a systematic decline in mass support for established political institutions, and a shift of focus toward individual concerns. (Inglehart 1997: 79)

Thus, in addition to an increasing reliance on computer-based technology within postindustrial societies, there is a concomitant increase in the
role of the individual and subsequent decrease in the importance of
bureaucratic structures. Although computers reduce the need for face-to-
face interaction between members of a society, the resulting increased levels of social isolation potentially alter the meaning and purpose of a
society's social institutions. As a result, social institutions such as education may be forced to redesign their teaching process to reflect the
changing demands and expectations of students relative to the core
knowledge level previously assumed necessary. Similarly, changes within
the occupational structure, the meaning of work as well as employer-
employee relations, are all undergoing fundamental reevaluation. Governments, at all levels, are also experiencing changes relative to those who
are governed. As these relationships are reexamined, potential changes in
the relationship between the individual and the state alter expectations of
who does what for whom. Consider, for example, the following statement:

It is time to integrate our understanding of the determinants of health and the
determinants of economic growth. Governments and their societies are mistaken
to concentrate on the economics of business cycles rather than the long-term forces
affecting economic growth, prosperity, and health and well-being. Fogel (1991) has
concluded that 50 percent of the economic growth in Britain since the Industrial
Revolution has been due to better nutrition of the population. A society that hand-
icaps large segments of its population during periods of major technological
change may be handicapping its future economic growth. (Frank and Mustard
1994: 15)

It is within this dynamic interinstitutional context that the health care
systems of the industrialized world are experiencing some of their most
profound challenges. For instance, one of the most formidable tasks of any
health system will be maintaining an increasingly aging population without increasing the cost of health care to the general public (Rathwell 1994;
Taylor-Gooby 1996). The development and application of costly technologies that extend life complicate this task. In addition, changes in the economic structure of societies will further differentiate populations on the
basis of social class position, age, sex, race, and ethnic origin, resulting in
an increased fragmentation of health-related opportunities and outcomes
within populations. Furthermore, all industrialized nations will be forced
to examine their commitment to the growth and application of medical
technology within health care.

Although medical technology expands the ability of health care
providers to improve the lives of ordinary citizens, it also fosters the emer-

gence of potentially adverse implications such as increased cost to the health care system (Bell 1989) as well as the medicalization of social life (Conrad 2000). Interwoven within these changes to the economic system are fundamental components of the health care system such as the delivery of health care and the mechanisms for financing. Thus, changing patterns of patient utilization, educational training of health professionals, and the cost of health care will redefine the health care workforce by altering current relationships such as the one between physician and patient. Acting in concert or individually, these changes will ultimately reshape health care systems throughout the industrialized world.

Relative to that process, Hsiao (1992) suggests three basic issues that all health care systems must address. They include "what proportion of its total resources are to be spent on health care?" Second, "how and by whom scarce health resources are to be allocated among programs, diseases, and regions?" Third, "nations must endeavor to obtain maximum efficiency in the production of health services" (614–615). These issues force an analysis of what constitutes a health care system, and they also address fundamental sociological explanations of such systems by examining the impact of differential economic outcomes relative to population arrangements, cultures, and social structures specific to each nation.

As evidenced earlier, health care systems are dynamic entities. Nevertheless, components of health care systems, such as their methods of financing and delivery, as well as regulatory procedures and educational requirements, are all criteria in constructing system typologies (see, for example, Elling 1984; Field 1980, 1989; Litman and Robins 1971; Roemer 1991; Twaddle 1996). As health care systems undergo change throughout the twenty-first century, the task will be to understand such change not only within the context of individual nations, but also as a representation of the intersection of political and economic forces relative to the cultural values of health care. It is within such a framework that this book is constructed.

The goal of this book is twofold. First, and most obvious, is to acquaint you with the significance of health care systems. Second, is to provide a framework for continued analysis of health systems worldwide. For example, given the current political realities in the United States, are alternative health care systems possible? Is the demonstrated ability of governmental bodies in all other industrialized nations to provide efficient and effective health care services and their delivery sufficient to warrant such an arrangement in the United States?

This book is intended for use within courses such as medical sociology, as well as public and health policy courses that address the macro-level issue of comparative health care systems. This book would work well as a supplement to my *Medical Sociology* text or function as the primary text within a comparative health care systems course. Although the primary audience for this book lies within the academic world, others will find the material, analysis, and recommendations of particular relevance as political and economic forces within the industrialized world attempt to force changes within health care communities around the world.

Finally, social scientists have an obligation to inform their audience of their biases. Relative to that point, this author, along with most Americans (see Navarro 1994: 195 for a list of some of the public opinion polls identifying support for a national health plan), supports the creation of a health care system that provides universal coverage for all citizens. The reasons for this position will become evident throughout the book.

## HEALTH CARE SYSTEMS DEFINED

It is generally agreed that all countries have some type of health care system, but there is less agreement regarding its definition. Consider the following definitions of what constitutes a health care system:

That aggregate of commitments and resources (human, cultural, political, and material) any society devotes to, or sets aside for, or invests into the "health" concern as distinguished from other concerns such as general education, defense, industrial production, communications, capital construction, and so on. (Field 1973: 764)

The health care system of a society can be broadly defined as a set of ideas, practices, and organizations which have been developed to deal with problems of health and illness in a society. (Lee 1982: 629)

A health care system may be defined as *the combination of health care institutions, supporting human resources, financing mechanisms, information systems, organizational structures that link institutions and resources, and management structures that collectively culminate in the delivery of health services to patients* [italics in original]. (Lassey, Lassey, and Jinks 1997: 3)

*The combination of resources, organization, financing, and management that culminates in the delivery of health services to the population* [italics in original]. (Roemer 1991: 31)

These definitions identify the conceptual range associated with health care system analysis. The definitions by Field (1973) and Lee (1982) offer broad interpretations that locate the health care system as part of the larger society, whereas the definitions by Lassey et al. (1997) and Roemer (1991) identify a highly specific set of structural arrangements located within the social system.

Integrating these two broad types of definitions, I would define a health care system as any combination of those components identified by a society that facilitates the provision of health and health care for its members. Although broad, such a definition allows for the specific cultural and historical development of health care systems. Such a definition, however, does not negate the importance of the components identified later in this chapter by Roemer, Elling, Light, or Field. Rather, this definition suggests that those components necessary or sufficient for creating any health care system depend on the characteristics of each society. A defined set of components may in fact exist within countries of the industrialized world, but it is presumptive to assume their universality, particularly within those nations that continue to experience severe economic problems and rely on traditional health care systems indigenous to the nation or specific populations. Given this definition and explanation, the next section examines a number of organizational arrangements associated with health care systems.

## HEALTH CARE SYSTEM ANALYSIS

Although societies differ in the arrangement of their health care system, they nonetheless have "a specific configuration of norms and values associated with numerous social institutions that constitute the health care system" (Matcha 2000: 366). Within this arrangement, a number of components are generally identified as constituting a health care system. This section identifies and discusses a number of arrangements that have been developed within the recent past. Although all offer unique explanations of health care systems, none are independently sufficient to explain all systems. For a succinct historical development of health care systems, see *The World Health Report 2000*.

The efforts of Roemer (1982, 1991) are perhaps best well known. Although societies differ regarding the importance of these components relative to their health care needs, their cross-cultural existence demonstrates their capacity to identify those functions considered essential within health care. According to Roemer, the primary components are management, resource production, economic support, organization of programs, and delivery of services. The purpose of each component and its subcategories is briefly discussed next.

The purpose of the *management* component is to explain how health care systems work: that is, how they are administered and regulated as well as the level of health system planning involved. This component provides an excellent entry into the comparative differences between health care systems. Consider, for example, the difference between the United States and other industrialized nations regarding the planning of the health care system. Within the United States, health care planning did not exist until the latter decades of the twentieth century. In other industrialized nations, planning at various governmental levels is an essential tool in cost control. However, even within other industrialized nations, the degree of planning varies.

*Resource production* refers to those areas within health care that are essential to its functioning. The subcategories within this component reflect these basic needs. For example, personpower refers to those individuals who provide necessary health care services. Facilities consist of hospitals, nursing homes, clinics, and other locations where health care services are provided. And, as Roemer (1991) notes, this would include the home of traditional healers. Commodities consist of those materials necessary for the treatment of patients. This ranges from hospital beds to pharmaceuticals. Finally, knowledge refers to that information necessary for the application of medical services. In other words, depending on the level of development, knowledge is represented through those methods of application and techniques known to the health care community in the prevention and treatment of diseases.

The *organization of programs* is essential within any health care system. How programs are organized depends on the type of health care system. For example, many countries have a Ministry of Health (MOH) within which all health services are organized. Features such as supply and demand organize systems that rely on the private health care market. For example, Americans living in rural areas or in poor neighborhoods of central cities have fewer health care options compared with suburban Americans. Physicians and related personnel and services are more likely to be located in those areas that can financially sustain their economic demands. Organizationally, other public agencies also provide health-related services. For example, social welfare services, services related to the workplace, the environment, or the social security of the elderly population, all represent programs beyond the scope of the MOH or the private health care market. Programs also include voluntary organizations that represent specific diseases, age populations (children, the elderly), health functions (Red Cross), religious beliefs, philanthropic foundations, and general social organizations. Enterprises refer to those arrangements, generally within the workplace, that offer health-related services to employees. Finally, all health care systems have a private proprietary market. The extent of this market is "inversely related to the strength of the minister of health" (Roemer 1991: 63).

The fourth component in Roemer's health care system is that of *economic support*. Its purpose is to identify methods for the financing of health care services. According to Roemer, although general tax revenues are used by most systems, they are particularly important sources of funding in those systems that employ ministers of health. Other funding mechanisms of health care systems include variations on social security. In other words, a percentage of employee wages is paid into a general fund used for health care benefits. Contributions by employers may or may not be matched. Some countries emphasize the use of voluntary insurance schemes whereby employees and/or employers contribute a defined amount per month into an insurance fund. An insurance company then pools the funds to cover the health care costs of its members. Other funding mechanisms include charitable donations and out-of-pocket payments by individuals and families.

The final component is the *delivery of services*. Roemer (1991) identifies three levels of delivery: primary, secondary, and tertiary. The World Health Organization (WHO) (1978) defines primary care as "Essential health care based on practical, scientifically sound and socially acceptable methods and technology made universally accessible to individuals and families in the community through their full participation and at a cost that the community and country can afford to maintain at every stage of their development in the spirit of self-reliance and self-determination" (3).

The World Health Organization further identified seven specific characteristics of primary health care. They range from preventive medical services to educating members of the community in the use and application of those services to the delivery of these services by health care professionals working as a team.

Roemer (1991) refers to secondary health care as "specialized ambulatory medical service, commonplace hospital care, care by nonmedical specialists, and general long-term care" (75). Finally, tertiary care includes those medical services that are extremely complex, require extensive technological intervention, and, as a result, are costly.

The health care system constructed by Roemer offers a detailed examination of those elements necessary for the provision of health care services. In contrast, others, such as Elling (1980), Field (1980), and Light (1994), incorporate not only the political and economic structures of society into their health care systems but also a number of specific characteristics such as the relationship between the physician and the state. These models are examined in detail next.

Elling (1980) offers a conceptualization of health care systems that incorporates multiple elements (blocks of variables) and their interrelated influence on health status. In this conceptualization, Elling addresses the importance of the social and cultural context within which the health system is located. Utilizing the concept of the ideal type, Elling (1980) argues "one can characterize an ideal health services system and hold it up against the realities of the health systems of the nations of the world to identify political-economic and other conditions which appear to support the ideal" (97).

Within this arrangement, Elling identifies the following broad areas: context, health planning apparatus, health services delivery system, and objectives. More specifically, the context refers to authority structures (political and economic) and their influence over health care arrangements. Elling is particularly concerned with class-based differences arising out of the organization of these authority structures. The second area, the health planning apparatus, is based on three key dimensions. These dimensions are first, the type of planning (systematic or pragmatic). Here, Elling refers to how planning is done. That is, is the planning rational or is it based on the beliefs of those engaged in the planning? The second dimension involves what he refers to as interrelatedness and inclusiveness. In other words, when planning occurs in other areas of society, does it factor in planning for health? According to Elling, the more interrelated and inclusive the planning, the better the outcome. The third dimension "is the access of the planning apparatus to the society's effective systems of social influence or power" (Elling 1980: 105). If those involved in health care planning do not have the power, implementation of health system needs is unlikely to be accomplished.

The third area in Elling's system is that of health services delivery system. Organizationally, this is the heart of Elling's argument. In particular, he believes a regionalized system would be the most effective arrangement for the delivery of health care. In support of a regionalized system, Elling offers a number of interwoven ideals associated with such a system.

Finally, Elling outlines specific objectives associated with his system. These objectives focus primarily on individual-level behavior such as satisfaction with care, but they also include issues such as knowledge and utilization of services.

Approaching health system development from a comparative perspective, Light (1994) constructed four models that represent ideal types. According to Light, these models are not representative of specific countries. Rather, actual systems depict combinations of these models. For comparative purposes, Light addresses eight specific features within each model. These points include key values and goals, image of the individual, power, key institutions, organization, division of labor, finance and costs, and medical education.

The *mutual-aid model* originated some four hundred years ago with the development of friendly societies or sickness funds. The purpose of such organizations was to provide funds for workers if they became ill or for families if the worker died. Initially these funds came from pooled resources provided by the workers. As the model developed, employers became the primary source of funding. This model emphasizes local control of services for members who are actively involved in the system. Because of the level of member involvement in this model, the state and the medical profession are secondary players in its management. Because of the emphasis on primary care, this model is likely to utilize a greater proportion of medical personnel other than physicians for the delivery of services.

The *state model* represents control of the health system by the government. The type of government is particularly important in terms of how health care is provided and for what reason. Autocratic governments can use health care as an indoctrination or reeducation tool against dissidents. Democratic governments are more likely to use health care as a means of controlling costs. Unlike the mutual-aid model, power in the state model resides in the state, rather than the consumer, and funding of the model is through general tax revenues. The power of the medical profession depends on the type of government. In other words, the medical profession is stronger in democratic governments but weaker under autocratic regimes. However, because of its interest in controlling costs, the state model is similar to the mutual-aid model in its emphasis on primary care.

Whereas the mutual-aid and state models view physicians as secondary or employees of the system, the *professional model* represents efforts to put physicians in charge of the system. That is, physicians are in control of health care decision making. The key value within the professional model is that physicians provide medical services to those patients capable of paying for them. Compared with the mutual-aid and state models, the professional model has a greater percentage of specialists. Financing of the health care system is through private sources rather than the government or sickness funds established by workers. The role of the state is minimal, and the profession of medicine is given free rein to design and implement methods that comply with its needs. As a result of minimal state intervention, greater inequalities exist within the professional model. These inequalities include differences in access to physicians as well as differences in access to health care opportunities. Because of the unwillingness of the state to regulate the cost of health care, the professional model is the most expensive model.

The *corporatist model* represents a synthesis of the previous models. According to Light, the corporatist model is a European construct. The government acts as an intermediary between all parties involved in health care. For example, health care costs and services are negotiated among employees, employers, physicians, and hospitals. In Germany, employers and employees contribute equally toward the payment of health care premiums.

Similarly, Field (1980) identifies a number of specific health-related criteria applied across a spectrum of ideal-type health care systems. The criteria include a general definition, position of the physician, role of professional associations, ownership of facilities, economic transfers, role of the polity, and prototypes. The ideal-type health care systems are anomic, pluralistic, insurance/social security, national health service, and socialized.

The *anomic* is characterized as a system within which physicians are solo practitioners paid directly by their patients. Government involvement in this system is minimal because control is vested primarily within the medical profession.

Although similar, the *pluralistic* type represents movement away from the power of physicians over the system. An example of this movement is the type of practice setting. In the pluralistic type of health care system, physicians are increasingly located in group, rather than solo practice. Furthermore, ownership of facilities has shifted from completely private to a mix of private and public, and payment for services is less direct.

The *insurance/social security* type represents a significant shift from the first two in that health care is guaranteed rather than a consumer good available only to those who can afford its cost. This shift acknowledges the increased influence of government in the health care arena. Accordingly, economic transfers are increasingly indirect, with health care costs covered through revenue enhancement (taxes) rather than direct consumer payment for services. Although physicians remain in solo and group practice, the strength of their professional organizations continues to diminish.

The *national health service* is characterized by even greater government involvement. In this case, health care is supported by the state. As a result, economic transfers are, for the most part, indirect, and the government is the primary owner of health care facilities. Physicians are in solo practice or members of medical organizations.

The *socialized* health care system is characterized by government ownership of health care facilities and physicians as employees of the state. Economic transfers are completely indirect, and control of the health care system is within the state.

These ideal types represent a continuum with the most entrepreneurial health care systems represented in the anomic and the most centralized located in the socialized model. Field identifies the United States and Western Europe in the nineteenth century as characteristic of the anomic type, and the former Soviet Union and Eastern bloc nations representative of the socialist type of health care. Given the recent political and economic changes within the former Soviet Union and Eastern bloc countries, the designation of socialist health care has undergone significant alteration.

These models of health care systems offer you a number of configurations that, when applied, differentiate between nations. Health care systems also provide a framework within which an analysis of differential outcomes within given populations can be examined and explained. According to Ertler et al. (1987), knowledge of health and disease and their distribution is essential to evaluating any health care system. For example, variation in health and disease patterns by age, sex, social class, and race and ethnicity provides the basis for an analysis of social, political, and economic influences on intra- and intercountry outcomes.

Health care systems offer medical sociology an analytic tool for assessing and explaining various health outcomes such as life expectancy, infant mortality, and so forth. Associated with these outcomes are the unique patterns of health care located within each country and their subsequent application through a uniquely structured delivery system appropriate to the economic and political needs and expectations of each society.

## HEALTH CARE SYSTEM MODELS

The classification of health care systems I employ in this book (i.e., entrepreneurial, Bismarck, Beveridge model, and state) is similar to the work of others (see, for example, Anderson 1989; Andrain 1998; Elling 1980; Field 1980; Graig 1999; Organization for Economic Cooperation and Development 1993; Roemer 1991). Examining the work of these authors reveals the various organizational arrangements that have been employed to represent the types of health care systems throughout the world. Given the various arrangements cited, it is obvious that agreement regarding an international classification system and location of countries does not exist.

As noted earlier, health care systems vary between nations for a variety of reasons. One of the most important reasons is that each system represents a unique set of cultural values. In addition to culture, political and economic institutions also influence health care systems (Unschuld 1979). The influence of these structures on the continuum of health care systems identified here is briefly addressed in this section. This continuum represents, in very broad terms, the range of health care systems in existence, regardless of their level of economic development. Although the purpose here is not to locate all countries within a particular health care system, Roemer (1991) offers a typology within which some 64 of the world's nations are identified.

The four types of health care systems identified in this chapter represent systems that range from the free market to state control of health care. Differences among these four types of health care systems are significant on a number of levels. In addition to the extent of governmental control over the provision and delivery of health care, these systems also differ in terms of control over professional obligations, methods of financing, as well as a host of other aspects associated with health care. For instance, one of the most often cited characteristics regarding health care costs is the amount spent per capita as well as health care spending as a percentage of gross domestic product (GDP). The United States remains the leader in both categories. According to the Organization for Economic Cooperation and Development (1999), the United States spent 14.0% of GDP on health care in 1998. By comparison, the percentage of GDP spent on health care in the other five countries examined in this book (Canada, United Kingdom, Germany, Sweden, and Japan) ranged from 6.9% of GDP in the United Kingdom to 10.6% in Germany. Also in 1998, total health care spending per capita in the United States was

$4,270. By contrast, total health spending per capita in the other countries presented in this book ranged from $1,450 in the United Kingdom to $2,400 in Germany (Organization for Economic Cooperation and Development 1999).

Although total health care spending increased within all of the selected countries, the rate of increase differs by country. For example, total health spending per capita increased 6.4% in Canada between 1990 and 1998. By comparison, per capita spending increased 20.1% in Germany, 31.9% in Japan, 21.7% in the United Kingdom, and 22.3% in the United States during the same period. By contrast, per capita spending on health care decreased by 2.2% in Sweden between 1990 and 1998 (Organization for Economic Cooperation and Development 1999). The implications of these differences will become increasingly evident throughout the remaining chapters of this book.

The following section offers a brief explanation of the four types of health care systems utilized throughout the world. The first, the entrepreneurial, is modeled on the characteristics of the private sector marketplace and characterized by the American health care system.

### Entrepreneurial Model of Health Care Systems

A strong private medical marketplace is characteristic of an entrepreneurial health care system (Roemer 1991). That is, the economics associated with health care provision and delivery occurs primarily between patients and health care providers. According to Roemer (1991), nations with an entrepreneurial health care system range from the economically developed United States, to the developing nations of Thailand, the Philippines, and South Africa to very poor nations such as Ghana, Bangladesh, and Nepal. Andrain (1998) also locates Canada within this system. Within the framework constructed in this book, as well as elsewhere, Canada is located within the Beveridge model.

What constitutes an entrepreneurial health care system? Andrain (1998) states that "the goals of efficiency, increased productivity, and cost containment take precedence over equal access to health services and equal treatment by medical personnel. To attain these goals, entrepreneurs support decentralization, competitive markets, and limited state intervention into the health care market" (19).

An entrepreneurial system is exemplified by the ongoing interplay between, on one hand, those engaged in the delivery of health care and those who control the methods of insuring citizens against the use of health care, on the other. Many of these issues are discussed in greater depth in chapter 2. However, because the United States represents the only industrialized nation with such an approach to health care, any explanation of the entrepreneurial health care system requires applying the American model as an example of advanced health care capabilities and the resultant consequences. For example, within recent years, the introduction of concepts such as *managed competition* and *managed care* has become one of the most significant components associated with the American entrepreneurial system. Managed competition involves a mixture of public and private funding of health care through a number of health providers who are "competing" for the pool of insurers. Enthoven and Kronick (1989) argue that under such a program "everyone not covered by an existing public program would be enabled to buy affordable subsidized coverage, either through their employers, in the case of full-time employees, or through 'public sponsors,' in the case of the self-employed and all others" (31).

Conceptually distinct from managed competition, managed care addresses an organizational effort to define how health care is provided. Although various definitions exist, Wholey and Burns capture the expanding implications associated with managed care. They define managed care organizations (MCOs) as *"organizations using administrative processes or techniques to influence the quality, accessibility, utilization, costs, and prices or outcomes of health services provided to a defined set of providers"* [italics in original] (2001: 219). Although various forms of managed care have been in existence for some time (e.g., HMOs), more recent efforts are effectively changing the relationship between physician providers and their patients. For instance, issues of health care and the associated costs are increasingly controlled by nonmedical decision makers rather than health-related personnel. These changes are creating increased divisiveness among those with vested interests in the health care system.

The entrepreneurial health care system in the United States has also been characterized by its inconsistency in providing and managing services for its citizens. Given the political nature of the American health care system, it is not surprising that the most significant organizational and structural efforts have been at the state, rather than the national, level. These efforts, however, illustrate one of the more difficult problems with the entrepreneurial system. That is, without national standards, differentiated health care opportunities and outcomes between states are likely. As a result, entrepreneurial health care systems such as the United States create inherently unequal health care opportunities for their citizens.

## Bismarck Model of Health Care Systems

France, Germany, Japan, the Netherlands, and Austria represent the social insurance, or Bismarck health system model. Whereas Roemer (1991) locates Canada within this model, I am following the arrangement offered by the Organization for Economic Cooperation and Development that places Canada within the Beveridge model (discussed next).

Although government (at various levels) is involved in financing health care, the social insurance model represents a partnership between the public and private sectors of the economy for the explicit purpose of ensuring health care coverage for its citizens. Thus a similarity between "Germany, the Netherlands, Japan, and France [is that they] all have occupation-based insurance programs to which employers and employees make joint financial contributions" (Andrain 1998: 59–60). Stated differently, "national health insurance,... is usually part of a general program of social security, also including old-age pensions, maternity benefits, unemployment compensation, disability insurance, and children's allowances" (Roemer 1991: 129). Countries with a social insurance health care system have, in the past, been able to control the overall growth in the cost of health care. Recently, however, health care costs have been rising in the selected countries at a faster rate when compared with selected countries with a Beveridge model of health care (see Table 1.1). Examining health care spending as a percentage of GDP between 1990 and 1998, countries with a social insurance type of health care system (Germany and Japan) experienced increases of 21.8% and 21.3%, respectively. During the same period of time, countries with a Beveridge model of health care (Canada and the United Kingdom) experienced increases of 1.09% and 15%, respectively, while Sweden recorded a 2.27% decrease. The American entrepreneurial health care system recorded an 11.1% increase (Organization for Economic Cooperation and Development 1999). One explanation for the increase within the German health care system is the reunification of East and West Germany in the early 1990s. As a result of the reunification, the East German health care system has been transformed from a state-run to a social insurance model.

Social insurance health care systems vary regarding the organizational structure and financing of the system. Because two of these systems (Ger-

Table 1.1
**Life Expectancy and Infant Mortality Rates: Selected Countries, 1999 (at birth)**

| Country | Life Expectancy[1] | Infant Mortality[2] |
|---|---|---|
| United States | 76.1 | 6.4 |
| Canada | 79.2 | 5.6 |
| Great Britain | 77.2 | 5.9 |
| Germany | 77.0 | 5.2 |
| Sweden | 79.2 | 3.9 |
| Japan | 80.0 | 4.1 |

[1]Number of deaths of children under 1 year of age per 1,000 live births in a calendar year.

[2]*Source:* U.S. Bureau of the Census, unpublished data from the International Data Base. U.S. Bureau of the Census (1998). *Statistical Abstract of the U.S. 1998,* 118th ed. Table 1345. Washington, DC: Government Printing Office.

many and Japan) are examined in considerable detail in later chapters, I do not spend time here discussing their arrangements.

In general, social insurance systems integrate public/private initiatives to ensure that all or most citizens have access to a basic package of health care services. Financing of social insurance systems also varies. For example, the German system is employment based, with employees and employers contributing an equal percentage of a worker's salary into a sickness fund. Although financing of health care is similar in the Netherlands, employers pay most of the insurance premium. Social insurance systems also formalize global budgeting in an effort to control health care spending. Global budgeting refers to the setting of financial spending limits on the delivery of health care services. In particular, global budgeting is applied to physician and hospital services. Generally, an agreed-upon spending limit is established between physicians and the government or delegated authorities charged with paying for the services. A similar agreement is established with hospitals.

One of the more limiting features of social insurance systems had been the lack of financial reserves for long-term care. Recently, however, many of these health care systems have been developing financing solutions (see detail in the following chapters). A second problem, not confined to the social insurance system, is the ongoing effort among the more politically conservative members of various governments to redefine the role of the state relative to health policy.

### Beveridge Model of Health Care Systems

The most significant differences between the Beveridge model and the social insurance system of health care are in terms of financing and the delivery of services. More specifically, the Beveridge model is more likely to rely on tax revenues for financing. With the emphasis for financing the health care system a government responsibility, health services and their access is more likely to be considered a right of citizenship. Thus, rather than rely on various financing and delivery schemes, the Beveridge model of health care systems is likely to locate the administration of the system within a Ministry of Health (MOH) office. The centralization of health care financing and services offers greater administrative savings and control over the delivery of services.

The Beveridge model of health care systems is located in countries such as Great Britain, Canada, Sweden, Norway, and Spain. Although each country has structured its health care system differently, the outcome within each is the same: all citizens have access to the system. Per capita health care costs are generally lower in countries with the Beveridge model. For example, per capita spending in the United Kingdom in 1998 was $1,450. In Sweden, Norway, and Spain, per capita spending was

$1,820, $2,090, and $1,240, respectively. By contrast, per capita spending on health care in the United States was $4,270. Health care spending as a percentage of GDP is also generally lower. In 1998, health care spending accounted for 6.9% in the United Kingdom and 8.6%, 7.5%, and 7.5% in Sweden, Norway, and Spain. By comparison, the United States spent 14.0% of GDP on health care (Organization for Economic Cooperation and Development 1999).

As with countries in the social insurance model, the Beveridge model has been the target of politically conservative efforts to relinquish state-level control of health care and allow for privatization of the system. This has been particularly evident in the United Kingdom. Beginning with Prime Minister Margaret Thatcher in the 1980s and continuing under Prime Minister John Major, the National Health Service (NHS) experienced a number of reform efforts (addressed in greater detail in chapter 4). Essentially, these efforts were to incorporate the work of American Alain Enthoven and his efforts at managed competition. The Swedish health care system has also been the target of politically conservative efforts to integrate an American-style for-profit arrangement within the government-sponsored system (see greater detail in chapter 6).

## State-Controlled Model of Health Care Systems

State-controlled health care systems were generally located in the former Soviet Union and the Eastern bloc countries such as Poland, Romania, and Czechoslovakia (now the Czech Republic and Slovakia). With the collapse of the communist state in the "Former Socialist Countries of Europe" (hereafter referred to as FSE), health care as well as economic and political systems is undergoing rapid transformation (see, for example, Angelus 1992 [Hungary]; Davidow 1996 [Soviet Union]; Field 1995 [Russia]; Mastilica 1992 [Yugoslavia]; Roemer 1994 [Poland and Hungary]; and Schreiber 1993 [Czechoslovakia]). With universal systems once financed by the state, many of the health care systems are being transformed into social insurance systems (Ensor 1993). As Ensor (1993) points out, this transformation is occurring for two reasons. First, physicians in these countries have been pushing for greater control of the health care system. Second, all of the countries are experiencing economic problems. Thus "payroll taxes in post-communist countries are probably one of the most secure funding sources" (Ensor 1993: 181). Prior to the collapse of the communist system, health care generally did not receive the level of funding necessary for adequate delivery of services to its residents. As a result, measures of a population's health (life expectancy and infant mortality) for the Soviet Union began to deteriorate after the 1960s. For example, Cockerham (1999) reports that mortality rates increased among "middle-aged, urban males in the most developed republics of the former Soviet Union" (20). Furthermore, life expectancy rates decreased for both males and females between 1979 and 1980 and 1991 and 1993 in a number of the former Soviet Republics (Cockerham 1999).

The future direction of health care systems in the former socialist countries of Europe is an area of interest (explored in greater depth in chapter 8). The general assumption is that health care systems within the FSE will converge (as they are now) toward a middle ground that incorporates a form of social insurance.

## CURRENT REALITIES

An overriding theme throughout this chapter is that although health care systems enjoy areas of similarity, they also differ, particularly with regard to the level and type of financing as well as the delivery of services. Essentially, health care systems reflect the beliefs of those with the economic and political power to influence their purpose and structure. As a result, the health of a population served by a particular health care system is a reflection, in part, of that system's effectiveness. Table 1.1 provides life expectancy and infant mortality rates for the six countries examined in this book.

The data in Table 1.1 indicate that life expectancy and infant mortality rates are not correlated with type of health care system. However, the data demonstrate the inefficiency of the American entrepreneurial system. Compared with the other countries in this book (and other industrialized nations in general), the American entrepreneurial health care system has the lowest life expectancy and highest infant mortality rates.

Whereas the data in Table 1.1 provide gross indicators of a nation's health, a recent World Health Organization (2000) study ranked overall health system performance. Although somewhat controversial, the report ranked the health care system in France as the best in the world. Among the countries in this book, Japan was ranked 10th, the United Kingdom 18th, Sweden 23rd, Germany 25th, Canada 30th, and the United States 37th. Based on the data, it is not possible to suggest a relationship between health care system and outcome performance among the selected countries, except that all countries identified here outperformed the American entrepreneurial health care system. The following chapters examine why.

## ROLE OF THE STATE

Health care systems throughout the world are experiencing political and economic pressures to reduce the influence of governmental control over the financing and delivery of services. Given the findings in the previous section, such pressure would appear unwarranted as increased government involvement in the health care system generally results in increased health outcomes for the population. For example, Hollingsworth, Hage, and Hanneman (1990) argue that increased state funding of medical services and state control of prices and personnel results in increased levels of efficiency and control of costs. Furthermore, "the ultimate responsibility for the overall performance of a country's health system lies with government, which in turn should involve all sectors of society in its stewardship. The careful and responsible management of the well-being of the population is the very essence of good government" (World Health Organization 2000: xiv).

Unfortunately, political systems are increasingly influenced by multinational market considerations that place profit from health-related services or products ahead of the best interests of the state or its citizens. It is expected that such a trend will have a deleterious effect on the aggregate health of nations.

These efforts are not confined to the industrialized world. As demonstrated earlier, the former socialist countries of Europe are experiencing significant changes in their political, economic, and health care institutions. Similarly, countries in the developing world are experiencing increasing economic pressures from organizations such as the World Bank to privatize their health care system (Sen and Koivusalo 1999). Developing nations also represent a wide range of state-level intervention in the health care system. For example, the Ghanaian health care system is entrepreneurial, whereas Cuba retains state control over health care. Health outcomes between the two countries are significant. According to the World Health Organization (2000) report cited earlier, the Cuban system is ranked 39th overall (the American system is ranked 37th) and Ghana at 135th. Health care spending in Cuba represents 6.3% of GDP, and it is 3.1% in Ghana. In Cuba, out-of-pocket expenditures as a percentage of total health expenditures are 12.5%; in Ghana, it is 53%. The data indicate that the type of health care system constructed by the state influences the distribution of health care costs as well as health outcomes within its population.

## THE HEALTH OF THE POPULATION BY AGE, SEX, SOCIAL CLASS, AND RACE AND ETHNICITY

An enduring problem within health care systems is the continued differentiation of health outcomes between population groups. For example, social class position, race, age, and sex influence morbidity rates among Americans (Matcha 2000). In addition, these variables influence not only a multiplicity of other health-related events but also the location of the individual within a particular society. This problem persists even within countries such as the United Kingdom where all citizens have had similar access to health services for over fifty years. Thus population health depends on more than access to health care services. All segments of a population must have access to those opportunities that will allow them to fully realize their social and economic potential. As with health, these opportunities differ by type of health care system. For example, the United States represents not only an entrepreneurial type of health care system but also an economic system wherein government assistance in the economic life of individuals is more limited than in the other industrialized countries examined in this book (see Abraham 1993 for an example of the failure of government health care assistance among the American poor). As a result of government policy, the United States is the most economically differentiated industrial society. The impact of these differences on population groups is addressed in the following chapters.

## OVERVIEW OF THE BOOK

The preceding sections offer you an introduction to health care systems in the world today. What is most evident is that no one health care system dominates the future direction of systems. Utilizing the continuum outlined by Anderson (1989), market-maximized countries (e.g., the United States) and market-minimized countries (e.g., the United Kingdom), it is possible to note movement toward applying similar system features because the industrialized nations are experiencing similar structural demands of their health care systems.

The next six chapters address health care systems in the United States, Canada, Great Britain, Germany, Sweden, and Japan. Throughout I examine the influence of the health care system on four critical variables: age, sex, race and ethnicity, and social class. The purpose of this approach is to compare the adequacy of each system relative to the most significant characteristics that locate individuals within their social system. I also address the historical and political basis for the current health care systems within the selected countries.

The final chapter explores the future of health care systems worldwide. I examine not only current arrangements within select health care systems, but also the potential for future configurations. Given the current political attitudes within the industrialized world today, changes within health care systems worldwide can be expected. Many of these changes will not be welcome because they represent efforts to deconstruct the influence of the state in the health affairs of nations. These efforts constitute a concerted effort by conservative politicians worldwide to privatize the financing and delivery of health care. Whether such efforts will succeed depends on the willingness of future generations to accept changes in the social contract between the state and its citizens relative to their health.

## CONCLUSION

This chapter introduced the diversity of thought associated with those health care systems currently found throughout the world. In the process, the chapter examined those components utilized in the analysis of health care systems as well as various models employed throughout the world. Examining the work of Roemer, Elling, Light, and Field, this chapter reported on the use of various system-level components to explain the diversity of health care systems worldwide. Secondly, this chapter examined four distinct models of health care. These models include the American entrepreneurial model; the social insurance, or Bismarck model (Germany, Japan); the Beveridge model (United Kingdom, Canada, Sweden); and the state-sponsored model previously employed by the former Soviet Union and Eastern bloc nations.

Throughout this chapter, I argued that the particular configuration of norms and values associated with a health care system represents the cultural beliefs of a particular nation. More specifically, I argued that the role of the state is crucial to identifying and implementing a health care system. In other words, the location of economic and political power within a nation is central to the emergence and maintenance of a health care system.

Finally, this chapter introduced the goals of the book. Although it is important to acquaint you with the importance of health systems, I believe it is equally necessary to provide a framework for analyzing the systems. To achieve these goals, the following chapters examine the impact of health care systems on those segments of the population differentiated on the basis of age, sex, social class, and race and ethnicity.

## REFERENCES

Abraham, Laurie Kay. 1993. *Mamma Might Be Better Off Dead: The Failure of Health Care in Urban America.* Chicago: University of Chicago Press.

Anderson, Odin W. 1989. *The Health Service Continuum in Democratic States: An Inquiry into Solvable Problems.* Ann Arbor, MI: Health Administration Press.

Andrain, Charles F. 1998. *Public Health Policies and Social Inequality.* New York: New York University Press.

Angelus, Tamas. 1992. "Consensus and Health Policy in Hungary." *The Journal of Medicine and Philosophy* 17: 455–462.

Bell, Susan E. 1989. "Technology in Medicine: Development, Diffusion, and Health Policy." In *Handbook of Medical Sociology,* 4th ed., ed. Howard E. Freeman and Sol Levine. Englewood Cliffs, NJ: Prentice-Hall.

Cockerham, William C. 1999. *Health and Social Change in Russia and Eastern Europe.* New York: Routledge.

Conrad, Peter. 2000. "Medicalization, Genetics, and Human Problems." In *Handbook of Medical Sociology,* 5th ed., ed. Chloe E. Bird, Peter Conrad, and Allen M. Freemont. Upper Saddle River, NJ: Prentice-Hall.

Davidow, Stephen L. 1996. "Observations on Health Care Issues in the Former Soviet Union." *Journal of Community Health* 21(1): 51–60.

Elling, Ray H. 1980. *Cross National Study of Health Systems*. Rutgers, NJ: Transaction Books.

———. 1984. "The Comparison of Health Systems in World-System Perspective." *Research in the Sociology of Health Care* 8: 207–226.

Ensor, Tim. 1993. "Health System Reform in Former Socialist Countries of Europe." *International Journal of Health Planning and Management* 8(3): 169–187.

Enthoven, Alain, and Richard Kronick. 1989. "A Consumer-Choice Health Plan for the 1990s: Part One." *New England Journal of Medicine* 320(1): 29–37.

Ertler, Wolfgang, H. Schmidt, J. M. Treyth, and H. Wintersberger. 1987. "The Social Dimensions of Health and Health Care: An International Comparison." *Research in the Sociology of Health Care* 5: 1–62.

Field, Mark G. 1973. "The Concept of the 'Health System' at the Macrosociological Level." *Social Science and Medicine* 7(10): 763–785.

———. 1980. "The Health System and the Polity: A Contemporary American Dialectic." *Social Science and Medicine* 14A(5): 397–413.

———. 1989. *Success and Crisis in National Health Systems: A Comparative Approach.* New York: Routledge.

———. 1995. "The Health Crisis in the Former Soviet Union: A Report From the 'Post-War' Zone." *Social Science and Medicine* 41(11): 1469–1478.

Fogel, Robert W. 1991. "The Conquest of High Mortality and Hunger in Europe and America: Timing and Mechanisms." In *Favorites of Fortune: Technology, Growth and Economic Development since the Industrial Revolution,* ed. David Landes, Parice Higgonet, and Nancy Rosovsky. Cambridge, MA: Harvard University Press.

Frank, John W., and J. Fraser Mustard. 1994. "The Determinants of Health from a Historical Perspective." *Daedalus* 123(4): 1–19.

Graig, Laurene A. 1999. *Health of Nations: An International Perspective on U.S. Health Care Reform,* 3rd ed. Washington, DC: Congressional Quarterly.

Hollingsworth, J. Rogers, Jerald Hage, and Robert A. Hanneman. 1990. *State Intervention in Medical Care: Consequences for Britain, France, and the United States, 1890–1970.* Ithaca, NY: Cornell University Press.

Hsiao, William C. 1992. "Comparing Health Care Systems: What Nations Can Learn from One Another." *Journal of Health Politics, Policy and Law* 17(4): 613–636.

Inglehart, Ronald. 1997. *Modernization and Postmodernization: Cultural, Economic, and Political Change in 43 Societies.* Princeton, NJ: Princeton University Press.

Lassey, Marie L., William R. Lassey, and Martin J. Jinks. 1997. *Health Care Systems Around the World: Characteristics, Issues, Reforms.* Upper Saddle River, NJ: Prentice-Hall.

Lee, Rance P. L. 1982. "Comparative Studies of Health Care Systems." *Social Science and Medicine* 16(6): 629–642.

Light, Donald. 1994. "Comparative Models of 'Health Care' Systems." In *The Sociology of Health & Illness: A Critical Perspective,* 4th ed., ed. Peter Conrad and Rochelle Kern. New York: St. Martin's Press.

Litman, Theodor J., and Leonard Robins. 1971. "Comparative Analysis of Health Care Systems—A Socio-Political Approach." *Social Science and Medicine* 5(6): 573–581.

Mastilica, Miroslav. 1992. "Health Inequalities and Health System Changes in the Former Yugoslavia." *International Journal of Health Sciences* 3(3–4): 195–203.

Matcha, Duane A. 2000. *Medical Sociology.* Boston: Allyn & Bacon.

Navarro, Vincente. 1994. *The Politics of Health Policy: The U.S. Reforms, 1980–1994.* Oxford: Blackwell.

Organization for Economic Cooperation and Development. 1993. *OECD Health Systems: Facts and Trends 1960–1991.* Health Policy Studies, No. 3. Paris, France.

———. 1999. *Health Data 99.* Paris, France.

Rathwell, Tom. 1994. "Health Care in Canada: A System in Turmoil." *Health Policy* 24: 5–17.

Roemer, Milton I. 1982. "Analysis of Health Services Systems—A General Approach." In *Reorienting Health Services: Application of a Systems Approach,* NATO Conference Series, Vol. 15., ed. Charles O. Pannenborg, Albert van der Werff, Gary B. Hirsch, and Kieth Barnard. New York: Plenum Press.

———. 1991. *The Countries.* Vol. 1 of *National Health Systems of the World.* New York: Oxford University Press.

———. 1993. "National Health Systems throughout the World." *Annual Review of Public Health* 14: 335–353.

———. 1994. "Recent Health System Development in Poland and Hungary." *Journal of Contemporary Health* 19(3): 153–163.

Schreiber, Vratislav. 1993. "The Medical Sciences in Czechoslovakia." *Technology in Science* 15(1): 131–136.

Sen, Kasturi, and Meri Koivusalo. 1999. "Health Care Reforms and Developing Countries—A Critical Overview." *International Journal of Health Planning and Management* 13(3): 199–215.

Taylor-Gooby, Peter. 1996. "The Future of Health Care in Six European Countries: The Views of Policy Elites." *International Journal of Health Services* 26(2): 203–219.

Twaddle, Andrew C. 1996. "Health System Reforms—Toward a Framework for International Comparisons." *Social Science and Medicine* 43(5): 637–654.

Unschuld, Paul U. 1979. "Comparative Systems of Health Care." *Social Science and Medicine* 13A(5): 523–527.

Wholey, Douglas R., and Lawton R. Burns. 2001. "Tides of Change: The Evolution of Managed Care in the United States." In *Handbook of Medical Sociology,* 5th ed., ed. Chloe E. Bird, Peter Conrad, and Allen M. Freeman. Upper Saddle River, NJ: Prentice-Hall.

World Health Organization. 1978. *Primary Health Care: Report of the International Conference on Primary Health Care.* Alma-Ata, USSR. Geneva, Switzerland.

———. 2000. *The World Health Report 2000. Health Systems: Improving Performance.* Geneva, Switzerland.

# CHAPTER 2

# The United States

American medicine, at this juncture, falls significantly short on each of the three basic goals that have guided health policy considerations over the past quarter-century—providing access in reasonable relationship to need; moderating the growth of medical care costs; and insuring uniformly high quality care.

(Mechanic 1994: 31)

## INTRODUCTION

The American health care system can best be understood as the result of the following characteristics: the availability of financial resources, a governmental structure that emphasizes decentralization, and a free market economy (Roemer 1986). Although these characteristics are not unique, they have been promulgated to a greater degree in the United States than other industrialized nations. The American health care system assumes that liberal economic principles such as competition and consumer sovereignty apply equally well to the provision and delivery of health services as they do to the purchasing of a computer or any other product. Although data have, for some time, demonstrated the fallacy of such an argument (see Fuchs 1993, for an analysis of why competition does not control health care costs), proponents of the current system continue to pursue increased application of these principles (Blendon and Edwards 1992). Health care, however, differs from other services. For example, Jonas (1998) argues that health care is part of the social/community market in which "broader individual, community, and social values" (3) are more important than private profit.

Health care also differs from liberal economic policy in terms of need. If I need a new car, I can shop around for the best deal at the price I am willing to pay. Regardless of the price range I am interested in, multiple automobile dealers exist for me to comparison shop. Health care is different from this and other market considerations in two respects.

One is that health care can be catastrophically costly. Much of the need for care is unpredictable, so it is vital for people to be protected from having to choose between financial ruin and loss of health.... The other peculiarity of health is that illness itself, and medical care as well, can threaten people's dignity and their ability to control what happens to them more than most other events to which they are exposed. (World Health Organization 2000: 24)

Proponents of liberal economic policy also argue "individuals are responsible for their own welfare, including health care" (Kronenfeld 1997: 13). Because of the emphasis on individual responsibility rather than coordinated planning, American health care has been referred to as a non-system (Enos and Sultan 1977). As a result, health care in the United States is represented by a multiplicity of actors with vested interests in their economic self-survival rather than the health of the system. For example, Angell (2000) argues that passage of a patient's rights bill could conceivably increase the number of uninsured Americans rather than improve the quality of care because health care as an employee benefit is not required. As a result, employers could discontinue offering such benefits if the cost became too high.

The entrepreneurial health care system in the United States is also characterized by its lack of genuine portability within a changing economic structure and its insensitivity to the insured. For the majority of Americans who have access to health care through the workplace (Altman, Reinhardt, and Shields 1998), the primary financial methods of entry are through health insurance and, increasingly, managed care organizations. Although access to health care is generally a workplace benefit, Americans cannot transfer their health care coverage from one job location to another. Although recent legislation (the Health Insurance Portability and Accountability Act of 1996) guarantees portability, it does not limit the rates a new insurer may charge if a worker or dependent has a preexisting condition (Reinhardt 1997). Thus workers are dependent on their employer, not only for a job, but also for maintaining health care benefits, if they exist.

Finally, the cost and structure of the American entrepreneurial health care system continues to create conditions that result in an increasing number of uninsured. The United States spends more per capita and as a percentage of GDP on health care than any other industrialized country. The National Center for Health Statistics (1999) reports preliminary figures for 1997 indicating health care consumed 13.5% of GDP, or $3,925 per capita. At the same time, Rhoades, Brown, and Vistnes (2000) report that some 43 million Americans do not have health insurance, with millions more inadequately insured. The number of uninsured Americans grew even throughout the relatively prosperous 1990s.

Schieber, Poullier, and Greenwald (1991) best summarize these problems when they state that "in comparison with other major industrialized countries, health care in the United States costs more per person and per unit of service, is less accessible to a large portion of its citizens, is provided at a more intensive level, and offers comparatively poor gross outcomes" (23). Thus the American entrepreneurial health care system begs the question: How can a system that spends so much per capita be so unequal? One response is that "the competitive marketplace is not designed to care for people who are not fortunate enough to have insurance" (Fletcher 1999: 1127). Ultimately, however, the answer lies in the American historical attitude toward health care.

## HISTORY OF THE AMERICAN HEALTH CARE SYSTEM

No defining moment signifies the inception of the American health care system. Rather, it evolved in conjunction with the norms and values of the larger culture. According to Iglehart (1992),

Over the past 200 years, the provision of medical care in the United States has been shaped by a variety of factors, including pragmatism, political imperatives, periodic health crises, the exercise of power by private interests, and a strong belief in limited government, individual freedom, and science and technology. (963)

Thus the historical development of the American health care system reflects not only cultural, but also political and economic influences that are characteristic of all health care systems (for an expanded historical presentation of American health care, see Matcha 2000).

In addition to their political, economic, and religious institutions, early-seventeenth-century European immigrants also brought with them current medical beliefs (Cassedy 1991). With few university-trained physicians, others, particularly religious leaders, were called on to minister to the medical as well as spiritual needs of the colonists (Dolan and Adams-Smith 1978). Although medicine was generally "dominated by quackery, mystical and superstitious beliefs, [and] home remedies" (Pfeiffer 1985: 103) throughout the seventeenth and eighteenth centuries, it became increasingly professionalized with the establishment of the first hospital and medical school in Philadelphia (see Gordon 1949: 13–15 for a list of significant medical events of the seventeenth and eighteenth centuries). Physicians also turned to European centers such as Paris and Edinburgh for training (Ackerknecht 1992). Placed within the social context of the time period, however, Shafer (1936) points out that at the time of the American Revolution, only 200 of the estimated 3,500 physicians in the colonies had a medical degree. It was during this time that the federal government first became involved in health care with the Act for the Relief of Sick and Disabled Seamen in 1798 (Kronenfeld 1997). The act allowed the government to tax seamen to cover the cost of their medical care.

At the beginning of the nineteenth century, the health of Americans remained relatively poor. Infant mortality rates remained high and life expectancy low. By the end of the century, however, the health of some Americans was improving (Leavitt and Numbers 1985). With the advent of the industrial revolution in the early nineteenth century also came increased urbanization and a minimal role for government (Duffy 1993). Throughout this period, the number of medical schools and students continued to increase. The growth of medical education did not result in increased professionalization because the quality of most medical schools and their students was suspect. For example, only one-fourth of the physicians passed the admissions test for the medical corps during the Civil War.

Following the Civil War, American medicine began to change. In particular, the status of the physician became increasingly distinct (Starr 1982). Medical education, however, was becoming polarized with schools such as Johns Hopkins, Harvard, and the University of Michigan providing quality medical education while proprietary institutions offered limited and inferior training to underqualified students. Shortly after the turn of the twentieth century, the Flexner Report provided the impetus for an increasing professionalization of physicians.

The twentieth century witnessed profound changes in the ability of medicine to treat disease and prolong life through medical technologies and pharmaceuticals. These advances, however, have come not only at a monetary cost, but a sociological one as well. For example, access and application of these biomedical advances has not been equal, as evidenced by the continued discrepancies between population groups in indicators such as life expectancy, infant mortality, morbidity/mortality rates, and health status (see, for example, Fiscella et al. 2000; Freeman and Payne 2000). These biotechnical advances have also created questions regarding the bioethics of living and dying.

Organizationally, the twentieth century witnessed significant changes in financing and delivery of health care services in the United States. For example, the 1930s witnessed the birth of Blue Cross as a hospital insurance system and Blue Shield to cover physician costs. Initially, the Blues were provided with a tax-exempt status because of their willingness to engage in community rating. More recently, however, that status has been revoked because their approach to insurance is "indistinguishable from those of commercial health insurers" (Navarro 1995: 191). Although available throughout the century, private health insurance became increasingly popular by mid-century.

In the 1970s, health maintenance organizations (HMOs) were touted as an alternative to traditional-based medicine. Most recently, managed care organizations (MCOs) and managed competition have dominated efforts to lower health care costs. All of these efforts have been within the private sector because governmental involvement in the health care system has historically been limited to the nonworking segments of the population. Furthermore, government involvement in health care distinguishes between "deserving" and "nondeserving" segments of the nonworking population. For example, in 1965, the passage of Medicare provided medical coverage to those aged 65 and over. Although an entitlement program funded by the federal government, Medicare coverage is extremely limited because it does not cover outpatient pharmaceuticals or long-term care, two expensive health-related components associated with the aging population. In contrast, Medicaid, also passed in 1965, provides means-tested health care coverage for the poor, regardless of age. Although Medicaid generally covers more health-related costs, individual states determine eligibility levels. If states set eligibility standards at extremely low-income levels, few will qualify for Medicaid, thus saving the state money. As a result, over half of the population living below the poverty line do not qualify for Medicaid. More recently, there has been an effort to ensure health care coverage of those children whose parents do not qualify for Medicaid, but are too poor to purchase health insurance. In addition to limited government-defined health care programs, the United States is the only member of the Organization for Economic Cooperation and Development (OECD) in which private funding of health care (55.9%) is greater than public (44.1%) monies (WHO 2000).

A number of efforts have also been made to create a national health care system in the United States. Kirkman-Liff (1997) identifies several periods throughout the twentieth century when efforts to reform American health care occurred. These efforts began in the first decade of the century when advocates for health care reform argued in support of a German insurance system. Opponents (those with a vested interest in maintaining a private system) were concerned with a loss of profits, and they were able to prevent implementation of any reform efforts. By the 1930s, the Committee on the Costs of Medical Care (CCMC) recommended the use of group insurance or taxation to cover the cost of medical care (CCMC 1932). Opponents again attacked any effort to change the current system. During World War II, agreement was reached among labor unions, industry, and the White House that health care benefits paid to workers would not be taxed. This agreement cemented the relationship between work and health care as a benefit.

In the latter 1940s, President Truman proposed a national health insurance program that was vilified as "socialized medicine" by the American Medical Association (see Laham 1993 for an analysis of health care reform during this period). By the mid-1960s, Medicare and Medicaid were enacted into law. Although important, these programs only intensified the role of both private insurance as a work-related benefit and government programs for dependent populations. By the 1970s, there was a concerted effort to marry the German insurance approach with health maintenance organizations (HMOs). This effort was lost when the Nixon White House became embroiled in the Watergate scandal.

The 1980s represented a period in which the relationship between work and health care as a benefit began to erode as larger companies self-insured and others engaged in experience rather than community rating (see Navarro 1994 for an analysis of the 1980s and early 1990s). The last attempt to create a unified health care system in the twentieth century occurred in 1993 when President Clinton proposed passage of the Health Security Act (The White House Domestic Policy Council 1993). Although this proposal was a "compromise between market-oriented and government-centered reform ideas" (Skocpol 1997: 15), the health insurance industry and radical right-wing politicians opposed it. A massive media campaign with the infamous Harry and Louise ads characterized the Health Security Act as a "big government" attempt to limit the health care of Americans. Although initially supported by an overwhelming percentage of the American population, the proposal quickly lost support and never came up for a vote in Congress.

The failure of these efforts has left the United States with an increasingly fragmented and multitiered health care system. Furthermore, the congressional elections of 1994 resulted in Republican control of both the Senate and House of Representatives. As a result, "interest in expanding access to medical care has declined" at the federal level (Iglehart 1995: 972). According to Kirkman-Liff (1997), the next attempt at health care reform will not occur for another 25 years. In the interim, Lemco (1994) offers this less than encouraging evaluation of what lies ahead for health care reformers:

The difficult task before American policymakers is to devise a system that is more efficient, cost effective, comprehensive, and universal while remaining sensitive to the desire by most Americans for a system that is consistent with their values and unique culture. It will be a formidable task. (273)

## FINANCING AND DELIVERY OF HEALTH CARE

One problem with the American system has been the fact that "proposals to reform the health care system focus on changing the way health care is financed, with little attention paid to how it is delivered, or to the distribution of services" (Mueller 1993: 169). Such lack of coordination, even within the reform movement, is indicative of how fragmented the American health care system has become.

With the demise of the Clinton Health Security Act in the early 1990s, expansion of managed care organizations (MCOs) has dominated the health care system. For example, the U.S. Bureau of the Census (1999) reports that the number of health maintenance organizations grew from 235 in 1980 to 572 in 1990 and 651 in 1998. Enrollment figures for the same years were 9.1, 33.0, and 64.8 million, respectively. MCOs, however, have been defining the health care industry since the mid-1960s (Wholey and Burns 2000). Increasingly, these organizations are for-profit, thus raising the specter of conflicting intentions of the organization (i.e., patient care versus stockholder expectations for profits).

Wholey and Burns (2000) point to the growing alphabet soup of health care organizational structures in the United States. For example, health maintenance organizations (HMOs) are defined as an organization "that accepts responsibility for the delivery of a predetermined range of necessary medical services to an enrolled population" (Luft 1998: 460–461). HMOs can be further delineated into a variety of models, including staff, group, network, and individual practice associations (IPAs). Managed care "is a much broader, and less well defined concept. It is often used to include, and sometimes primarily to mean HMOs, although it usually includes systems that may not meet the specific regulatory requirements of certain public agencies" (Luft 1998: 460–461).

The increased utilization of managed care organizations impacted the cost of health care in the 1990s. Although premium increases were minimal during much of the 1990s, costs again began to rise in the latter years of the decade. These increases are problematic because managed care organizations have already eliminated excess fat out of their systems. The potential result will be not only significant premium increases for consumers but also an expanding base of uninsured Americans. These dual responses reflect the American emphasis on the private sector as the primary method of financing health care. Without significant reform of the health care system, the cost of providing health care will continue to escalate. Efforts to change the system incrementally by making it more efficient and/or competitive will only exacerbate its financial problems. Compounding this problem is America's unwillingness to commit national resources (tax revenues) toward financing individual access. As a result, the American health care system is reaching a financial watershed regarding its ability to continue affordable coverage to its citizens. Examining the data in Table 2.1, health insurance coverage by age indicates that less than 60% of young adults (19–29) had private health insurance coverage in the first half of 1998, and almost one-third of those aged 19 to 24 and 27.4% of those aged 25 to 29 were uninsured.

**Table 2.1**
**Health Insurance Coverage of the Civilian Noninstitutionalized Population:**
**Percentage by Type of Coverage and Selected Population Characteristics,**
**United States, first half of 1998**

Percentage Distribution

| Population Characteristic | Private | Public Only | Uninsured |
|---|---|---|---|
| Total | 68.6% | 15.6% | 15.8% |
| Total under age 65 | 70.4 | 11.8 | 17.8 |
| Age in Years | | | |
|   Under 4 | 59.4 | 27.6 | 13.1 |
|   4-6 | 61.6 | 24.3 | 14.1 |
|   7-12 | 66.6 | 18.7 | 14.7 |
|   13-17 | 69.7 | 14.1 | 16.2 |
|   Total under 18 | 65.1 | 20.3 | 14.7 |
|   18 | 67.6 | 12.3 | 20.1 |
|   19-24 | 59.1 | 9.1 | 31.8 |
|   25-29 | 64.5 | 8.1 | 27.4 |
|   30-34 | 71.1 | 8.1 | 20.8 |
|   35-54 | 78.2 | 6.8 | 15.1 |
|   55-64 | 76.2 | 10.9 | 12.9 |
|   18-64 | 72.8 | 8.1 | 19.1 |
|   65 and over | 55.3 | 43.8 | 0.9 |
| Employment Status[a] | | | |
|   Employed | 79.4 | 4.5 | 16.1 |
|   Not Employed | 52.4 | 31.7 | 15.9 |
| Sex | | | |
|   Male | 68.9 | 13.7 | 17.4 |
|   Female | 68.4 | 17.4 | 14.2 |
| Race/Ethnicity | | | |
|   Total Hispanic | 46.9 | 21.3 | 31.8 |
|   Total Black | 50.2 | 29.2 | 20.6 |
|   Total White | 75.7 | 12.1 | 12.2 |
|   Total Other | 61.0 | 19.8 | 19.2 |
|   Hispanic male | 47.1 | 19.0 | 33.9 |
|   Black male | 50.0 | 26.8 | 23.2 |
|   White male | 76.1 | 10.4 | 13.6 |
|   Other male | 61.0 | 19.3 | 19.7 |
|   Hispanic female | 46.7 | 23.7 | 29.6 |
|   Black female | 50.4 | 31.3 | 18.3 |
|   White female | 75.4 | 13.8 | 10.9 |
|   Other female | 60.9 | 20.3 | 18.8 |
| Marital Status[b] | | | |
|   Married | 78.8 | 9.6 | 11.6 |

More specifically, the data illustrate significant differences in insurance coverage on the basis of race/ethnicity and marital status. According to the data, 31.8% of Hispanics are uninsured, compared with 20.6% of blacks and 12.2% of whites. Interestingly, 46.9% of Hispanics and 50.2% of blacks have private health insurance. By comparison, 75.7% of whites report health coverage through private health insurance. Given the con-

**Table 2.1 (continued)**

| | | | |
|---|---|---|---|
| Widowed | 50.7 | 43.1 | 6.2 |
| Divorced | 62.2 | 18.2 | 19.6 |
| Separated | 50.6 | 22.1 | 27.2 |
| Never Married | 61.6 | 12.2 | 25.7 |
| Metropolitan Statistical Area | | | |
| MSA | 69.8 | 15.0 | 15.3 |
| Non-MSA | 64.0 | 18.2 | 17.8 |
| Census Region | | | |
| Northeast | 70.8 | 16.5 | 12.7 |
| Midwest | 76.1 | 12.4 | 11.4 |
| South | 64.8 | 16.4 | 18.8 |
| West | 65.0 | 17.0 | 18.1 |

[a]Includes persons with unknown employment status and marital status.

[b]For individuals age 16 and over.

Note: Percentages may not add to 100 because of rounding.

*Source:* Center for Cost and Financing Studies, Agency for Healthcare Research and Quality: Medical Expenditure Panel Survey Household Component, 1998. Rhoades, J., E. Brown, and J. Vistnes. *Health Insurance Status of the Civilian Noninstitutionalized Population: 1998.* Table 1. Rockville (MD): Agency for Healthcare Research and Quality: 2000. MEPS Research Findings No. 11. AHRQ Pub. No. 00-0023.

tinued growth in minority populations, the data do not offer hope for the future. Similar differences exist on the basis of marital status: 78.8% of married Americans have private insurance coverage, but only 50.7% of widowed and 50.6% of separated Americans claim similar coverage.

Examining the relationship between the workplace and insurance coverage illustrates what could be characterized as the fundamental problem with the American health care system. That is, among workers aged 19 to 24, only 59.2% had private health insurance coverage in the first half of 1996, and 35.5% were uninsured. Although the percentage of workers aged 25 to 29 with private health insurance increased, over 23% remained uninsured. Female workers were more likely to have private health insurance than male workers. By race and ethnicity, over 82% of white workers had private health insurance, whereas only two-thirds of black workers and 57.6% of Hispanic workers had private health insurance. Females, regardless of race or ethnic origin, were more likely to have private health insurance than males, and male workers, regardless of race or ethnic origin, were more likely to be uninsured. In particular, 43.5% of employed Hispanic males were uninsured (Monheit and Vistnes 1997).

Further examination of health insurance coverage among American workers reveals the impact of the work environment. For example, as the size of the workplace decreases, the percentage of workers with private health insurance decreases and the percentage of uninsured increases.

**Table 2.2**
**Medical Care Benefit Coverage and Average Monthly Employee Contributions, 1980–1997**
**[Covers full-time employees in private nonfarm establishments. Based on a sample survey of establishments; for details, see Source and headnotes, Tables 709 and 710]**

| | Establishment Size | | | | |
|---|---|---|---|---|---|
| | Medium and Large | | | Small | |
| | 1980 | 1991 | 1997 | 1990 | 1996 |
| Percentage of full-time employees participating | 97 | 83 | 76 | 69 | 64 |
| PERCENTAGE DISTRIBUTION OF PARTICIPATING FULL-TIME EMPLOYEES | 100 | 100 | 100 | 100 | 100 |
| Traditional fee for service[1] | (NA) | 67 | 27 | 74 | 36 |
| Preferred provider organization[2] | (NA) | 15 | 40 | 13 | 35 |
| Health Maintenance Organization[3] | (NA) | 17 | 33 | 14 | 27 |
| Other | (NA) | --- | 1 | --- | 2 |
| Individual coverage | | | | | |
| Employee contributions not required | (NA) | 49 | 31 | (NA) | 48 |
| Employee contributions required | 26 | 51 | 69 | 42 | 52 |
| Family Coverage | | | | | |
| Employee contributions not required | (NA) | 31 | 20 | (NA) | 24 |
| Employee contributions required | 46 | 69 | 80 | 67 | 75 |
| AVERAGE MONTHLY EMPLOYEE CONTRIBUTION (dol.) | | | | | |
| Total | (NA) | 27 | 39 | 25 | 43 |
| Non-HMO[4] | (NA) | 26 | 42 | 25 | 43 |
| HMO | (NA) | 29 | 34 | 25 | 41 |
| Family coverage | | | | | |
| Total | (NA) | 97 | 130 | 109 | 182 |
| Non-HMO[4] | (NA) | 92 | 132 | 104 | 181 |
| HMO | (NA) | 118 | 126 | 135 | 182 |

—Represents zero. NA Not Available.

[1]These plans pay for specific medical procedures as expenses are incurred.

[2]Groups of hospitals and physicians that contract to provide comprehensive medical services at prearranged prices. To encourage use of organization members, the health plan limits reimbursement rates when participants use nonmember services.

[3]Includes federally qualified and other HMOs that deliver comprehensive health care on a prepayment rather than fee-for-service basis.

[4]Includes traditional fee-for-service plans, preferred provider plans, and exclusive provider organization plans.

*Source:* U.S. Bureau of Labor Statistics, *News*, USDL 98-240, June 15, 1998; *News*, USDL 99-02, January 7, 1999; and earlier releases.

*Source:* United States Census Bureau. *Statistical Abstract of the United States, 1999.* Table 186. Washington, DC: Government Printing Office.

As the number of full-time workers with health insurance coverage through their employer declines (see Table 2.2), so will affordable health care. For others, especially those with Medicaid coverage or the uninsured, access to health care is generally limited to hospital emergency rooms or health centers, if available. According to recent testimony before the U.S. Senate Subcommittee on Public Health and Safety, the associate director of Health Financing and Public Health Issues stated that 40% of Health Center patients were uninsured. Thirty-three percent of the uninsured were Hispanic, and 25% were African Americans. At the same time, health center revenue will decline as states are allowed to reduce their Medicaid reimbursement levels (General Accounting Office 2000).

In addition to a decreasing percentage of full-time employees with health care coverage, those who are covered are increasingly in a managed care organization and required to make greater employee contributions for care. This is particularly true for employees in small companies, which are also less likely to offer health care as a benefit of employment.

A similar relationship exists between hourly wages and private insurance coverage and the likelihood of being uninsured. For instance, although only 48.8% of workers who earn $5 an hour have private health insurance, 96.8% of workers earning $20 or more per hour are covered. Finally, compared with workers who do not belong to a union, workers with membership in a union are much more likely to have private health insurance (93.6% and 76.3%, respectively) (Monheit and Vistnes 1997).

The preceding data illustrate the problem of connecting health care benefits to the workplace when such benefits are not mandatory. With continued realignment within the workplace toward nonunionized, smaller service-oriented companies, the number of uninsured workers is expected to increase, thus polarizing the workforce and creating greater competition for a decreasing percentage of positions with benefits. Those workers and their dependents for whom health care is not a benefit will continue to swell the ranks of the uninsured. The impact of an economically constructed health underclass is problematic not only in terms of an inability to afford the cost of health care, but also to a diminished incentive to work. Continued increases in the number of uninsured and a concomitant decrease in the number of insured could destabilize the current financing structure of the American health care system.

The American health care system continues to be financed through a patchwork of private third party entities that includes insurance companies and managed care organizations as well as government-sponsored programs. Operationally, this means that monies are collected through a number of sources that include "payroll taxes; enrollee premiums; federal and state general revenues" (Chollett 1993: 24). According to the data in Table 2.3, health care expenditures, regardless of the source, have

Table 2.3
**Personal Health Care Expenditures, by Source of Payment, 1980–1996, and Projections, 1998–2005**
[In billions of dollars (217.0 represents $217,000,000,000). The health spending projections for 1998 to 2005 were based on the 1996 release of the national health expenditures (NHE). Subsequent release of the NHE may not be consistent with these projections and should not be substituted for the 1996 historic estimates.]

Projections

| SOURCE OF PAYMENT | 1980 | 1990 | 1998 | 2000 | 2005 |
|---|---|---|---|---|---|
| Total | 217.0 | 614.7 | 998.2 | 1,124.2 | 1,603.2 |
| Out-of-pocket payment | 60.3 | 144.4 | 183.7 | 206.9 | 276.6 |
| Third party payments | 156.8 | 470.3 | 814.5 | 917.3 | 1,326.5 |
| Private health insurance | 62.0 | 206.7 | 321.6 | 372.8 | 550.8 |
| Other private funds | 7.8 | 21.3 | 35.5 | 40.8 | 56.4 |
| Government | 87.0 | 242.3 | 457.3 | 503.7 | 719.3 |
| Federal | 63.4 | 177.6 | 369.4 | 296.2 | 562.3 |
| State, local | 23.6 | 64.7 | 96.9 | 107.5 | 157.0 |
| Medicare[1] | 36.4 | 109.3 | 223.6 | 243.0 | 342.1 |
| Medicaid[2] | 24.8 | 71.4 | 154.9 | 175.9 | 266.5 |

[1]Medicare expenditures come from federal funds.

[2]Medicaid expenditures come from federal and state and local funds.

*Source:* U.S. Health Care Financing Administration, Office of the Actuary, "TO2a;" published September 28, 1998; http://www.hcfa.gov/stats/NHE-Pro/tables/to2a.htm.

*Source*: U.S. Bureau of the Census. *Statistical Abstract of the United States, 1999.* Table 172. Washington, DC: Government Printing Office.

increased significantly since 1980 and are projected to continue their upward spiral.

According to the data in Table 2.3, total health care expenditures are projected to increase by 639% between 1980 and 2005. More specifically, during the same 25-year period, private health insurance contributions are expected to increase by 788% and government expenditures by 726%. Among government expenditures, Medicare increased by 839% and Medicaid by 975%. These increases do not reflect the impact of the aging baby boomer population on the health care system, particularly Medicare. Beginning in 2011, baby boomers will begin turning 65, resulting in an ever-increasing need for health care services.

Given our knowledge of greater health care utilization among older populations and a shrinking pool of employer-provided health care benefits, health care financing is of particular concern because current projections place the financial collapse of Medicare at 2025, well before the entire baby boomer generation is eligible for its benefits. If the window of opportunity to significantly reform health care financing closes, the current system will be unable to provide those services necessary to maintain a culturally and chronologically diverse population without devastating their financial resources.

These data reinforce the argument that the American health care system is experiencing a number of structural deficiencies. For example, compared with other industrialized nations, the cost of providing health care services for shorter periods of time is greater in the United States. Furthermore, American financing schemes are less efficient because of their inability to guarantee all citizens coverage and access to health care services. The only financing mechanism that approximates universal coverage of its intended population is Medicare. Medicare, however, does not guarantee universal access to all necessary health services. Rather, individuals are expected to purchase so-called medi-gap insurance to ensure access to services not provided through Medicare. This discrepancy illustrates the problem with an entrepreneurial approach to health care. That is, American health policy does not connect access to coverage. The argument is made that co-pays or deductibles will limit individuals from excessive utilization of health services. Thus access to health services is considered an individual rather than a societal responsibility. Given the unequal distribution of income and wealth in the United States, it is not surprising that access to and distribution of those health care benefits necessary for maintaining a healthy life is also unequal.

## Physicians

Prior to the twentieth century, most American physicians had little formal training. Although attempts were made to improve the profession through licensure and improved quality of existing medical schools, these efforts generally failed. Shortly after the turn of the twentieth century, however, the American Medical Association (AMA) surveyed the existing medical schools. Rather than release their findings (which suggested closing many of the schools), the AMA commissioned the Carnegie Foundation to conduct a similar survey. The foundation hired Abraham Flexner, who eventually visited all of the medical schools in the United States. The recommendations laid out in the Flexner Report were more negative than the unpublished AMA report. Flexner recommended upgrading some institutions to the Johns Hopkins model, and he also argued for the closure of most medical schools in the United States (Starr 1982). Although such Draconian measures were never officially implemented, many of the medical schools closed shortly after the report was made public. As a result, the Flexner Report had a significant impact on medical education and the profession of medicine. With the declining number of medical schools and, subsequently, students, the status of the remaining students increased as the quality of medicine improved within the existing institutions.

The status of physicians was also enhanced by the expansion of medical technologies throughout the twentieth century. Thus physicians currently rank at the top of the occupational prestige ladder in the United States.

In addition to an improved occupational prestige, American physicians also experience considerably higher levels of earnings than their Canadian, Japanese, or European counterparts. In 1992, American physicians had a gross income of $182,000. By comparison, gross income (in American dollars) for physicians in Germany was $104,700; Canada $100,781; Japan $48,022; the United Kingdom $42,826 (1999); and Sweden $39,082 (Organization for Economic Cooperation and Development 2000). However, the average number of patient visits per week to American physicians has been decreasing while the average hours in patient care per week have increased (U.S. Bureau of the Census 2000).

The number of physicians in the United States continues to increase. In 1980, there were 467,700 active physicians in the United States. By 1998, there were 777,900 (U.S. Bureau of the Census 2000). Recently, however, the number of students applying to medical schools has been decreasing. The declining attraction of medicine is, in part, the result of diminishing autonomy and a changing professional status accorded physicians within the rapidly expanding managed care organizations. For example, McKinlay and Marceau (2001) point to the middle of the twentieth century as the "golden age" of doctoring, whereas the end of the twentieth century reflects the decline of medicine as a profession.

### Hospitals

The hospital system in the United States is characteristic of the American health care system. In other words, many hospitals offer the newest medical technologies available in the fight against disease and death. At the same time, many hospitals are experiencing financial difficulties because an increasing number of patients are unable to afford these services. Rosenberg (1987) best characterizes the American hospital as "an institution that reproduces values and social relationships of the wider world yet manages at the same time to remain isolated in its particular way from the society that created and supports it" (4).

The American hospital system also reflects the problems of delivering health care services. Although the number of hospital beds per 100,000 population is comparable with other industrialized nations, the average daily cost per patient bed is the most expensive in the world. Thus the greater cost of care is not the result of an excessive supply of beds in the United States relative to other industrialized nations. Americans also have shorter hospital stays when compared to most other industrialized nations. However, costs per patient day and stay are generally higher in the United States than other industrialized countries, indicating greater application of medical technologies and other services (Organization for Economic Cooperation and Development 1994). Within the United States, for example, the number of hospitals decreased from 7,156 in 1975 to 6,097 in 1997. The number of beds also declined from 1,465,828 in 1975 to 1,035,390 in 1997. The only area where the number of hospitals and hospital beds has increased is within the for-profit sector. Relative to other types of hospitals, for-profit hospitals have also experienced a greater percentage increase in the number of employees. Utilization of hospital beds also depends on type of ownership. Governmental and nongovernmental nonprofit hospitals averaged around 64% occupancy in the mid-1990s. During the same period, however, occupancy rates in for-profit facilities averaged just 50% (National Center for Health Statistics 1999).

Although American hospitals will survive, they will experience considerable changes as they accommodate the decreasing availability of funds for the humanitarian provision of health care services. Interconnected to these changes are the continued advancements associated with medical technologies and their possible outcomes for hospitals (see, for example, Stevens 1991). These technologies are a factor in increasing hospital expenses, but they do not completely explain the aberrant levels associated with American facilities.

## CURRENT REALITIES AND THE ROLE OF THE STATE

We previously examined the historical framework within which the current American health care system is situated. This section addresses its current realities. More specifically, here, among other things, we analyze the health of the population on the basis of four sociological variables: age, sex, social class, and race and ethnicity. For purposes of international comparison, these variables are explored relative to all health care systems presented in the next five chapters. But first, what is the current state of health care in America?

Unequivocally, the American health care system is in a state of disrepair. With the failure of the Clinton Health Security Act, health care policy has become increasingly politicized and polarized. On the one hand, health care reform advocates continue to advance scenarios that envision variations on existing systems (such as Canada or Germany). For example, McDermott (1994), a member of the House of Representatives and a physician, has consistently advocated for a single-payer system. On the other hand, opponents of health care reform continue to successfully locate their maintenance of a private, for-profit system within the framework and ideology of an antigovernment argument. The result is an increasing commodification of the American public as health care fodder with health data providing the ideological grist for the media and political battlegrounds within which the war over the direction of the health care system is being fought. In the process, the role of the state has become increasingly pivotal in determining the direction and financing of the health system.

The following statement illustrates why the federal government has experienced such difficulty controlling the health care system:

That the federal government accounts for only 33% of national health expenditures moderates the extent to which the federal government is able to regulate health affairs and why it must be responsive to the concerns of the state governments, private hospitals, medical associations, health insurance companies, and others who have a role in the health system. (Raffel and Raffel 1997: 264)

Given the American penchant for a decentralized political system and a competitive marketplace, the historical lack of government involvement in the health care system is not surprising. According to Jacobs (1993), government involvement in health care did not occur until "the 1920s, [and then] in an indirect, nonsalient way: it encouraged nonstate institutions to organize and finance the country's health care" (54). Such arrangements, however, have created a policy environment that requires the development of innovative financing and delivery methods: for example, the development of insurance programs such as Blue Cross in the 1930s, and, more recently, efforts to include other nonworking populations into government-sponsored health initiatives. Nationwide, individual states have developed Children's Health Insurance Programs under Title XXI of the Social Security Act. The Child Health Plus program in New York State enrolled over 140,000 children as of August 1997 with an additional 422,000 children eligible for the benefits, based on family income of 200% or less of the federal poverty guidelines. At the time, it was the "largest State-subsidized health insurance program in the nation" (New York State Department of Health 2000).

In addition to funding initiatives targeting dependent populations, recent health care reform efforts have been located at the state level. For example, a referendum on the Fall 2000 ballot in Massachusetts would have required the state to provide universal health care by 2002 ("White Coat Rebels" 2000: A3). Throughout the 1990s, various state-level initiatives have been advanced. Differences among states, however, are significant. As Iglehart (1994) notes, "the difference in health care spending among states is greater than the difference between spending in the United States and in some other industrialized nations" (75).

The latest federal effort to provide universal health care coverage for all Americans is also at the state level. House Bill 4075 was introduced in the House of Representatives on March 23, 2000. This bill states the following:

1. Access to health care is a basic right protected by the Constitution of the United States.
2. Each State should determine the minimum level of health services to be provided within each State.
3. Any health care system operated by a State that does not provide access to health care to all citizens of each State is in violation of the Fourteenth Amendment to the Constitution of the United States.
4. Federal funds may not be employed to support State health care systems that are unconstitutional. (House of Representatives, 106th Congress, 2nd Session 2000, Health Care Access Assurance Act of 2000: 2)

If this bill were passed in its original form, the United States would potentially have 50 different versions of universal coverage. Although flawed, this bill recognizes that if the federal government is unwilling to ensure universal access to health care to the general population, then responsibility for such an effort lies with state governments. Unfortunately, the devolving of government responsibility for the health of the population creates the potential for increased differentiation of health outcomes among various segments of the population. As the following section indicates, health outcomes already differ on the basis of age, sex, and race and ethnicity, as well as social class.

## THE HEALTH OF THE POPULATION BY AGE, SEX, SOCIAL CLASS, AND RACE AND ETHNICITY

In the aggregate, the health of the American population relative to other industrialized nations is poor. Compared with the other five countries in this book, the United States ranks last in life expectancy for both males and females and infant mortality. Internationally, the United States ranked 19th in female life expectancy, 25th in male life expectancy, and 25th in infant mortality in 1995 (National Center for Health Statistics 1999).

Disaggregated, the health of the American population is highly variable, indicating the influence of sex, age, social class, and race and ethnicity on disease patterns and health outcomes. Thus, when proponents of the current system tout the phrase that the United States has the best health care system in the world, they are referring to a system that exists for a declining number of Americans.

The remainder of this section examines the increasing differentiation of health problems and outcomes on the basis of age, sex, social class, and race and ethnicity in the United States. Much of the information in the following sections is drawn from chapters 3 through 5 in Matcha (2000).

## Age

All industrialized nations are experiencing a demographic shift as their populations age. In the United States, the population aged 65 and over currently represents approximately 13% of the total population. It is projected to increase to 18.7% by 2025. More importantly, the oldest-old are currently the fastest growing segment of the population. In 1970, they constituted 1.8% of the population. By 2025, they will increase to 4.3%. By comparison, the other five nations examined in this book will all have a greater percentage of their population over the ages of 65 and 80 when compared with the United States. For example, it is estimated that by 2025, 26.7% of the population in Japan will be aged 65 and over, and 9.3% will be age 80 or over (U.S. Bureau of the Census 1992).

The importance of this demographic shift relative to the health care system is that morbidity and mortality rates are related to age. That is, as we age, death and disease rates increase. The consequence to the health care system is an ever-increasing cost as more services are provided to a growing number of individuals within the age categories most at risk. Examining death rates for diseases of the heart, cerebrovascular diseases, and malignant neoplasms from the National Center for Health Statistics (1999), death rates among Americans begin to increase during early to mid-teenage years and continue to do so throughout the remainder of the life cycle. Similarly, morbidity rates are also related to age. For example, those aged 65 and over experience more than twice the number of restricted activity days than do those below age 65 (see Matcha 2000). Compared with younger individuals, older persons generally experience a greater prevalence of chronic conditions. According to Spillman and Lubitz (2000), the average medical care cost for people aged 65 until their death is $164,505. Given the increased morbidity rates, it is not surprising that older persons also have the highest rate of office-based physician visits (U.S. Bureau of the Census 1999). Furthermore, persons aged 65 and over are more likely than those below age 65 to define their health status as fair or poor.

## Sex

As with age, rates of disease and health outcomes are differentiated on the basis of sex. In addition, mortality rates also differ between men and women. The data in Table 2.4 illustrate these differences between 1970 and 1997, as well as differences on the basis of age and race. Mortality rates increase with age, particularly among those aged 55 to 64, and mortality rates also differ between white and black Americans, regardless of sex and

**Table 2.4**
**Death Rates by Sex, Race, and Select Ages, 1970–1997**
**[Number of deaths per 100,000 population in specified groups.**
**See headnote, Table 130]**

| Sex, year, and race | Under 1 year old | 45-54 years old | 65-74 years old | 75-84 years old | 85 years old and over |
|---|---|---|---|---|---|
| MALE[1] | | | | | |
| 1970 | 2,410 | 959 | 4,874 | 10,010 | 17,822 |
| 1980 | 1,429 | 767 | 4,105 | 8,817 | 18,801 |
| 1990 | 1,083 | 610 | 3,492 | 7,889 | 18,057 |
| 1995 | 844 | 599 | 3,285 | 7,377 | 17,979 |
| 1996 | 828 | 574 | 3,233 | 7,250 | 17,548 |
| 1997 | 807 | 546 | 3,195 | 7,141 | 17,559 |
| WHITE | | | | | |
| 1970 | 2,113 | 883 | 4,810 | 10,099 | 18,552 |
| 1980 | 1,230 | 699 | 4,036 | 8,830 | 19,097 |
| 1990 | 896 | 549 | 3,398 | 7,845 | 18,268 |
| 1995 | 718 | 535 | 3,199 | 7,321 | 18,153 |
| 1996 | 683 | 516 | 3,158 | 7,206 | 17,871 |
| 1997 | 682 | 493 | 3,130 | 7,122 | 17,890 |
| BLACK | | | | | |
| 1970 | 4,299 | 1,778 | 5,803 | 9,455 | 12,222 |
| 1980 | 2,587 | 1,480 | 5,131 | 9,232 | 16,099 |
| 1990 | 2,112 | 1,261 | 4,946 | 9,130 | 16,955 |
| 1995 | 1,591 | 1,273 | 4,611 | 8,779 | 16,729 |
| 1996 | 1,748 | 1,191 | 4,432 | 8,615 | 16,006 |
| 1997 | 1,614 | 1,101 | 4,271 | 8,178 | 15,887 |
| FEMALE[1] | | | | | |
| 1970 | 1,864 | 517 | 2,580 | 6,678 | 15,518 |
| 1980 | 1,142 | 413 | 2,145 | 5,440 | 14,747 |
| 1990 | 856 | 343 | 1,991 | 4,883 | 14,274 |
| 1995 | 690 | 328 | 1,986 | 4,883 | 14,292 |
| 1996 | 680 | 323 | 1,979 | 4,868 | 14,445 |
| 1997 | 648 | 316 | 1,959 | 4,828 | 14,530 |
| WHITE | | | | | |
| 1970 | 1,615 | 463 | 2,471 | 6,699 | 15,980 |
| 1980 | 963 | 373 | 2,067 | 5,402 | 14,980 |
| 1990 | 690 | 309 | 1,924 | 4,839 | 14,401 |
| 1995 | 572 | 294 | 1,925 | 4,831 | 14,639 |
| 1996 | 558 | 291 | 1,929 | 4,827 | 14,643 |
| 1997 | 536 | 286 | 1,904 | 4,803 | 14,739 |
| BLACK | | | | | |
| 1970 | 3,369 | 1,044 | 3,861 | 6,692 | 10,707 |
| 1980 | 2,124 | 768 | 3,057 | 6,212 | 12,367 |
| 1990 | 1,736 | 639 | 2,866 | 5,688 | 13,310 |

**Table 2.4 (continued)**

| 1995 | 1,342 | 619 | 2,824 | 5,840 | 13,472 |
|------|-------|-----|-------|-------|--------|
| 1996 | 1,444 | 610 | 2,787 | 5,776 | 13,399 |
| 1997 | 1,350 | 583 | 2,710 | 5,592 | 13,501 |

[1]Includes other races not shown separately.

*Source:* U.S. National Center for Health Statistics, *Vital Statistics of the United States,* annual; *National Vital Statistics Reports* (NVSR) *(formerly Monthly Vital Statistics Report);* and unpublished data.

*Source:* U.S. Bureau of the Census. *Statistical Abstract of the United States, 1999.* Table 131. Washington, DC: Government Printing Office.

chronological age (see Krieger and Fee 1994 for an example of the interrelationships among sex/gender, race/ethnicity, and social class on women's health).

The data in Table 2.4 indicate that although the health of Americans has improved (declining death rates), there are large differences between African Americans and white Americans, regardless of sex. These racial differences are discussed in greater detail in the next section.

Health differences between males and females have been attributed to a number of causes, including biological, environmental, and social. For example, males have higher rates of death than females, regardless of age. It has also been argued that because men are more likely to smoke, drink alcoholic beverages, and engage in riskier behavior than women, they are likely to experience more disease and increased mortality rates.

### Social Class

As noted earlier, the social class position of respondents is generally not one of the primary variables associated with health-related research in the United States. The following statement, however, underscores the significance of social class position; "in study after study socioeconomic status emerges as one of the most important influences on mortality and morbidity" (Angell 1993: 126) (see also Feinstein 1993; Rice 1991). Additional evidence identifies a linear relationship between social class position and fair or poor health status for whites, blacks, and Hispanics (National Center for Health Statistics 1999) (see Dutton 1986 for a visual description of the relationship between being poor and health status). Furthermore, health outcomes are influenced by the interrelationship of social class and race and ethnic identity. Regardless of level of education, "blacks and Hispanics usually have worse health than whites" (Krieger and Fee 1993: 64).

Not surprisingly, access to health care is related to social class position (Davis 1991). For example, as hourly wages increase, the percentage of

workers who are uninsured decreases. Furthermore, changing employment patterns are shifting workers into smaller firms and self-employment,
areas of the economy with the highest rates of uninsured workers. Thus
health care in the United States is becoming more a responsibility of the
individual than a benefit associated with the workplace. This will only
exacerbate those economic distinctions that currently exist between social
categories and compound their already tenuous relationships.

As this section indicates, a person's age, sex, race and ethnicity, and
social class individually, and in combination, define health access and consequent outcomes. These variables consistently support the argument that
within the fragmented and profit-motivated American health care system,
the patient's social position matters. It is within this context that the final
section explores how health care is currently financed and delivered in the
United States.

### Race and Ethnicity

As with age and sex, health care use and outcomes in the United States
also vary on the basis of one's race and ethnic heritage (see, for example,
Smith 1998). As the data in Table 2.4 indicate, black Americans fare less
well than white Americans. Interestingly, the United States is again
unique relative to other industrialized nations in that it reports health outcomes based on race, whereas others utilize social class. Although minority populations generally earn less than whites, it is an egregious
assumption to assume that racial and ethnic identity and social class are
interchangeable variables. Examining racial and ethnic differences in
health status, Williams and Collins (1995) point out that relative to whites,
Hispanics are similar, blacks have higher death rates, and Asian and
Pacific Islander Americans have lower death rates. Similarly, Campbell
(1989) points out that during the 1980s, "white infant mortality improved
by approximately 14 percent, while the American Indian rate eroded by 12
percent" (131).

Researchers have identified a number of explanations for the differences in mortality between blacks and whites (see Rogers 1992 for a list of
medically related causes for the differential in life expectancy between
blacks and whites). For example, regardless of social class position,
"blacks often have worse health indicators than whites" (Navarro 1990:
1240). More specifically, LaVeist (1993) argues, "when the black-white
infant mortality disparity is examined within smaller geographic units, a
more complex relationship between race and infant mortality emerges"
(54). Thus, according to LaVeist, poverty, racial residential segregation,
and black political empowerment influence infant mortality rates. The
level of poverty and geographic location were also cited relative to excess
mortality among African Americans (Geronimus et al. 1996).

Sorlie and others (1993) found that among Hispanics, mortality rates were lower than among non-Hispanics. They also report variations in mortality rates by location of birth within the Hispanic population. However, they caution that if Hispanics acquire those risk factors associated with chronic diseases, their mortality rates "are likely to increase" (2468).

## CONCLUSION

American health care is the most expensive in the world, and, among the industrialized nations, the least accessible. The entrepreneurial American system is characteristic of the larger economic structure that argues for broad-based competition as the cure-all for containing costs. This chapter noted, however, that purchasing health care is not like buying an automobile or computer. When purchasing an automobile or computer, the buyer has a number of purchasers and various option packages that can be added or deleted, depending on an individual's economic position. In health care, the ability to "shop around for the best deal" does not exist. Health care services are also not priced depending on one's economic position. Thus, if I need heart surgery, I cannot elect to purchase surgery A rather than surgery B because B is too expensive.

The American entrepreneurial health care system differs from the other models discussed in this book in two major respects: its lack of universal coverage and the number of uninsured. Although numerous health reform efforts throughout the twentieth century have garnered considerable public support, they have not been politically successful. As a result, the American health care system remains mired in a highly politicized struggle between various segments of society supporting differing alternatives, on the one hand, and those supporting greater competition and other liberal economic approaches applied to the health care system, on the other. Because employers are not required to provide health care as a workplace benefit, the number of employees left without affordable access to services has increased significantly, even during the economic boom period of the mid- to late 1990s. In addition, managed care organizations (particularly for-profit companies) have increased their role within the health care delivery system. As a result, access to services potentially depends on decision making that weighs the cost of a service relative to the profit-making needs of the organization.

Similar to other industrialized nations, differential health outcomes on the basis of age, sex, social class, and race and ethnicity exist in the United States. However, gross indicators of the population's health locate the United States ranking last in life expectancy and infant mortality when compared with the other countries in this book. Thus health care in the United States mirrors the broader socioeconomic differences that characterize the country. In other words, for some, the American health care system is the best in the world if they can afford it. For an increasing number of uninsured and underinsured, however, the American health care system represents the worst possible scenario: knowing the medical technology necessary to save or improve one's life exists, but unable to access the services because they are unaffordable.

## REFERENCES

Ackerknecht, Edwin H. 1992. *A Short History of Medicine*, rev. ed. Baltimore: Johns Hopkins University Press.

Altman, Stuart H., Uwe E. Reinhardt, and Alexandra E. Shields. 1998. "Healthcare for the Poor and Uninsured: An Uncertain Future." In *The Future U.S. Healthcare System: Who Will Care for the Poor and Uninsured?* ed. Stuart H. Altman, Uwe E. Reinhardt, and Alexandra E. Shields. Chicago: Health Administration Press.

Angell, Marcia. 1993. "Privilege and Health—What Is the Connection?" *New England Journal of Medicine* 329(2): 126–127.

———. 2000. "Patients' Rights Bills and Other Futile Gestures." *New England Journal of Medicine* 342(22): 1663–1664.

Blendon, Robert J., and Jennifer N. Edwards. 1992. "Health Care Cost Containment in 1997: Two Scenarios." In *Reforming the System: Containing Health Care Costs in an Era of Universal Coverage*, ed. Robert J. Blendon and Tracey Stelzer. New York: Faulkner & Gray's Healthcare Information Center.

Campbell, Gregory R. 1989. "The Political Epidemiology of Infant Mortality: A Health Crisis among Montana American Indians." *American Indian Culture and Research Journal* 13(3&4): 105–148.

Cassedy, James H. 1991. *Medicine in America: A Short History.* Baltimore: Johns Hopkins University Press.

Chollett, Deborah J. 1993. "Health Care Financing in Selected Industrialized Nations: Comparative Analysis and Comment." In *Trends in Health Benefits.* U.S. Department of Labor. Pension and Welfare Benefits Administration. Washington, DC: Government Printing Office.

Committee on the Costs of Medical Care. 1932. *Medical Care for the American People. The Final Report.* No. 28. Chicago: University of Chicago Press.

Davis, Karen. 1991. "Inequality and Access to Health Care." *Milbank Quarterly* 69(2): 253–273.

Dolan, John P., and William N. Adams-Smith. 1978. *Health and Society: A Documentary History of Medicine.* New York: Seabury Press.

Duffy, John. 1993. *From Humors to Medical Science: A History of American Medicine.* Urbana: University of Illinois Press.

Dutton, Diana B. 1986. "Social Class, Health, and Illness." In *Applications of Social Science to Clinical Medicine and Health Policy*, ed. Linda H. Aiken and David Mechanic. New Brunswick, NJ: Rutgers University Press.

Enos, Darryl D., and Paul Sultan. 1977. *The Sociology of Health Care: Social, Economic, & Political Perspectives.* New York: Praeger.

Feinstein, Jonathan S. 1993. "The Relationship between Socioeconomic Status and Health: A Review of the Literature." *Milbank Quarterly* 71(2): 279–322.

Fiscella, Kevin, Peter Franks, Marthe R. Gold, and Carolyn M. Clancy. 2000. Inequality in Quality: Addressing Socioeconomic, Racial, and Ethnic

Disparities in Health Care." *Journal of the American Medical Association* 283(19): 2579–2584.

Fletcher, Robert H. 1999. "Who Is Responsible for the Common Good in a Competitive Market?" *Journal of the American Medical Association* 281(12): 1127–1128.

Freeman, Harold P., and Richard Payne. 2000. "Racial Injustice in Health Care." *New England Journal of Medicine* 342(14): 1045–1047.

Fuchs, Victor R. 1993. *The Future of Health Policy.* Cambridge, MA: Harvard University Press.

General Accounting Office. 2000. *Health Care Access: Programs for Underserved Populations Could Be Improved.* Testimony before the Subcommittee on Public Health and Safety, Committee on Health, Education, Labor, and Pensions. U.S. Senate. March 23.

Geronimus, Arline T., John Bound, Timothy A. Waidmann, Marianne M. Hillemeier, and Patricia B. Burns. 1996. "Excess Mortality among Blacks and Whites in the United States." *New England Journal of Medicine* 335(21): 1552–1558.

Gordon, Maurice Bear. 1949. *Aesculapius Comes to the Colonies: The Story of the Early Days of Medicine in the Thirteen Original Colonies.* Ventnor, NJ: Ventnor Publishers.

House of Representatives. 2000. Health Care Access Assurance Act of 2000. 106th Congress, 2nd Session. Washington, DC.

Iglehart, John K. 1992. "The American Health Care System: Introduction." *New England Journal of Medicine* 326(14): 962–967.

———. 1994. "Health Care Reform: The States." *New England Journal of Medicine* 330(1): 75–79.

———. 1995. "Republicans and the New Politics of Health Care." *New England Journal of Medicine* 332(14): 972–975.

Jacobs, Lawrence R. 1993. *The Health of Nations: Public Opinion and the Making of American and British Health Policy.* Ithaca, NY: Cornell University Press.

Jonas, Steven. 1998. *An Introduction to the U.S. Health Care System,* 4th ed. New York: Springer.

Kirkman-Liff, Bradford. 1997. "The United States." In *Health Care Reform: Learning from International Experience,* ed. Chris Ham. Buckingham: Open University Press.

Krieger, Nancy, and Elizabeth Fee. 1993. "What's Class Got to Do with It? The State of Health Data in the United States Today." *Socialist Review* 23(1): 59–82.

———. 1994. "Man-Made Medicine and Women's Health: The Biopolitics of Sex/Gender and Race/Ethnicity." *International Journal of Health Services* 24(2): 265–283.

Kronenfeld, Jennie Jacobs. 1997. *The Changing Federal Role in U.S. Health Care Policy.* Westport, CT: Praeger.

Laham, Nicholas. 1993. *Why the United States Lacks a National Health Insurance Program.* Westport, CT: Praeger.

LaVeist, Thomas A. 1993. "Segregation, Poverty, and Empowerment: Health Consequences for African Americans." *Milbank Quarterly* 71(1): 41–64.

Leavitt, Judith Walzer, and Ronald L. Numbers. 1985. *Sickness & Health in America: Readings in the History of Medicine and Public Health,* rev. 2nd ed. Madison: University of Wisconsin Press.

Lemco, Jonathan. 1994. "Conclusion." In *National Health Care: Lessons for the United States and Canada,* ed. Jonathan Lemco. Ann Arbor: University of Michigan Press.

Luft, Harold S. 1998. "Medicare and Managed Care." *Annual Review of Public Health* 19: 459–475.

Matcha, Duane A. 2000. *Medical Sociology.* Boston: Allyn & Bacon.

McDermott, Jim. 1994. "The Case for a Single-Payer Approach." *Journal of the American Medical Association* 271(10): 782–784.

McKinlay, John B., and Lisa D. Marceau. 2001. "Addendum 2000: The End of the Golden Age of Doctoring." In *The Sociology of Health and Illness: Critical Perspectives,* ed. Peter Conrad. New York: Worth.

Mechanic, David. 1994. *Inescapable Decisions.* New Brunswick, NJ: Transaction.

Monheit, A.C., and J.P. Vistnes. 1997. "Health Insurance Status of Workers and Their Families: 1996." *MEPS Research Findings No. 2.* AHCPR Pub. No. 97–0065. Agency for Health Care Policy and Research. Rockville, MD; Washington, DC: Government Printing Office.

Mueller, Keith J. 1993. *Health Care Policy in the United States.* Lincoln: University of Nebraska Press.

National Center for Health Statistics. 1999. *Health, United States, 1999: With Health and Aging Chartbook.* Hyattsville, MD: Public Health Service.

Navarro, Vincente. 1990. "Race or Class versus Race and Class: Mortality Differentials in the United States." *The Lancet* 336: 1238–1240.

———. 1994. *The Politics of Health Policy: The U.S. Reforms, 1980–1994.* Oxford: Blackwell.

———. 1995. "The Politics of Health Care Reform in the United States, 1992–1994: A Historical Review." *International Journal of Health Services* 25(2): 185–201.

New York State Department of Health. 2000. www.health.state.ny.us/nysdoh/chplus/cplus-1htm.

Organization for Economic Cooperation and Development. 1994. *The Reform of Health Care Systems: A Review of Seventeen OECD Countries.* Paris, France.

———. 2000. *OECD Health Data 2000. A Comparative Analysis of 29 Countries.* Paris, France.

Pfeiffer, Carl J. 1985. *The Art and Practice of Western Medicine in the Early Nineteenth Century.* Jefferson, NC: McFarland.

Raffel, Marshal W., and Norma K. Raffel. 1997. "The Health System of the United States." In *Health Care and Reform in Industrialized Countries,* ed. Marshall W. Raffel. University Park: Pennsylvania State University Press.

Reinhardt, Uwe. 1997. "Employer-Based Health Insurance: R.I.P." In *The Future U.S. Healthcare System: Who Will Care for the Poor and Uninsured?* ed. Stuart H. Altman, Uwe E. Reinhardt, and Alexandra E. Shields. Chicago: Health Administration Press.

Rhoades, J.E. Brown, and J. Vistnes. 2000. *Health Insurance Status of the Civilian Noninstitutionalized Population: 1998.* Agency for Healthcare Research and

Quality: 2000. MEPS Research Findings No. 11. AHRQ Pub. No. 00–0023. Washington, DC: Government Printing Office.

Rice, Dorothy P. 1991. "Ethics and Equality in U.S. Health Care: The Data." *International Journal of Health Services* 21(4): 637–651.

Roemer, Milton I. 1986. *An Introduction to the U.S. Health Care System.* New York: Springer.

Rogers, Richard G. 1992. "Living and Dying in the U.S.A.: Socioeconomic Determinants of Death among Blacks and Whites." *Demography* 29(2): 287–303.

Rosenberg, Charles E. 1987. *The Care of Strangers: The Rise of America's Hospital System.* Baltimore: Johns Hopkins University Press.

Schieber, George J., Jean-Pierre Poullier, and Leslie M. Greenwald. 1991. "Health Care Systems in Twenty-Four Countries." *Health Affairs* 10(3): 22–38.

Shafer, Henry Burnell. 1936. *The American Medical Profession, 1783 to 1850.* New York: Columbia University Press.

Skocpol, Theda. 1997. *Boomerang: Health Care Reform and the Turn against Government.* New York: W.W. Norton.

Smith, David Barton. 1998. "Addressing Racial Inequalities in Health Care: Civil Rights Monitoring and Report Cards." *Journal of Health Politics, Policy and Law* 23(1): 75–105.

Sorlie, Paul D., M. S. Backlund, N. J. Johnson, and E. Rogot. 1993. "Mortality by Hispanic Status in the United States." *Journal of the American Medical Association* 270(20): 2464–2468.

Spillman, Brenda C., and James Lubitz. 2000. "The Effect of Longevity on Spending for Acute and Long-Term Care." *New England Journal of Medicine* 342(19): 1409–1415.

Starr, Paul. 1982. *The Social Transformation of American Medicine.* New York: Basic Books.

Stevens, Rosemary. 1991. "The Hospital as a Social Institution, New-Fashioned for the 1990s." *Hospital and Health Services Administration* 36(2): 163–173.

The White House Domestic Policy Council. 1993. *The President's Health Security Plan: The Clinton Blueprint.* New York: Times Books.

U.S. Bureau of the Census. 1992. International Population Reports, P25, 92–3, *An Aging World II.* Washington, DC: Government Printing Office.

———. 1999. *Statistical Abstract of the United States.* Washington, DC: Government Printing Office.

———. 2000. *Statistical Abstract of the United States.* Washington, DC: Government Printing Office.

"White-Coat Rebels Urge Health Care Reform." 2000. *Albany* (New York) *Times Union,* June 11, p. A3.

Wholey, Douglas R., and Lawton R. Burns. 2000. "Tides of Change: The Evolution of Managed Care in the United States." In *Handbook of Medical Sociology,* 5th ed., ed. Chloe E. Bird, Peter Conrad, and Allen M. Freemont. Upper Saddle River, NJ: Prentice-Hall.

Williams, David R., and Chiquita Collins. 1995. "U.S. Socioeconomic and Racial Differences in Health: Patterns and Explanations." *Annual Review of Sociology* 21: 349–386.

World Health Organization. 2000. *The World Health Report. Health Systems: Improving Performance.* Geneva, Switzerland.

# CHAPTER 3

# Canada

What Canadians refer to as "Medicare" is in fact a series of provincial insurance plans, cost-shared with the federal government under the terms of the Canada Health Act, which requires that all Canadians must have "reasonable access," without direct charges, to all hospital and medical services deemed "medically necessary."

(Leatt and Williams 1997: 20)

## INTRODUCTION

The Canadian health care system is often incorrectly referred to as "socialized medicine." In reality, the system is more appropriately understood as socialized insurance (Evans 1993). The system is also referred to as National Health Insurance (NHI). Organizationally, the Canadian system has been located in various models. For example, Roemer (1991) identifies the Canadian system within the welfare-oriented model similar to that of Germany, France, and Japan, and Andrain (1998) places it with the United States in the entrepreneurial model. The Organization for Economic Cooperation and Development (OECD) locates the Canadian system within the Beveridge model along with other countries such as the United Kingdom, Sweden, Norway, Spain, Denmark, Australia, New Zealand, Portugal, and Italy. According to Angus (1998), health care systems in the Beveridge model are characterized by "universal coverage for the country's residents, financing derived by national general taxes, and some form of national ownership/control of the factors of production" (26). Relative to this book, I am following the OECD classification and locating Canada within the Beveridge model.

The Canadian health care system consists of "an interlocking set of ten provincial and two territorial health insurance schemes. Each is universal and publicly funded" (Organization for Economic Cooperation and Development 1994: 103). The provision of care in the national health insurance program, or Medicare, originates at the provincial and territorial level providing coverage for most health care needs without out-of-pocket expense incurred by patients (Rozek and Mulhern 1994).

Currently, each province negotiates reimbursement rates with groups representing service providers (i.e., hospitals and physicians). Doctors bill and are reimbursed by the province for services rendered, and hospitals operate within global budgets arrived at through negotiation with the provincial government. Thus the concept of a "single payer" system exists at the provincial, not the national, level. The Canadian health care system is unique relative to other industrialized nations, in that a parallel private health care system is not allowed to exist. In defense of such an arrangement, Evans (1993) argues that "private insurance for the whole population is impossible in a competitive marketplace, because insurers cannot cover the poor and the ill and remain competitive" (17). However, the majority of residents (through their employer) have a "voluntary, supplemental private insurance for services not covered by the public program" (Chollet 1993: 11) (e.g., prescription drugs, dental care, out-of-country services, and so forth) (Rozek and Mulhern 1994). These supplemental health programs also account for the most rapid growth rates in health care expenditures (Colvin 1994). The publicly funded system controls expenditures by limiting the application of medical technologies and the use of a "single payer" administrative structure (Iglehart 1989).

The limitation of medical technologies is evident when the number of computer tomography (CT) scanners and magnetic resonance imaging (MRI) units per million population in Canada is compared with the United States. In 1997, there were 8.2 CT scanners and 1.8 MRI units per million in Canada compared with 13.7 CT scanners and 7.6 MRI units per million population in the United States (Organization for Economic Cooperation and Development 2000).

In terms of performance, the World Health Organization has ranked the Canadian health care system 30th in the world (World Health Organization 2000). According to basic health statistics such as life expectancy, Canadians rank among the healthiest in the world. (See Table 1.2 for a comparison of life expectancy and infant mortality rates among the six nations discussed in this book.)

Politically, the Canadian health care system is experiencing its worst crisis since its inception. As some political leaders in Canada continue efforts to dismantle a health care system that has been described as "an enormous achievement, and light years ahead of the U.S.'s wildly expensive, out-of-control, profit-laden non-system" (Livingston 1998: 267), there has been a loss of public confidence (Iglehart 2000a). This crisis is the result of decreased funding at the national and provincial levels and an effort to regionalize services. In particular, conservative provincial governments in Ontario and Alberta are leading the drive for a two-tiered privatized system (see, for example, the Canadian Health Coalition 2000a for an analysis of the current crisis). Efforts to discredit the Medicare program are supported by organizations such as Citizens for Better Medicare, which has been running advertisements in the United States depicting the Canadian system as unable to provide necessary services to its citizens ("How Many Canadian Seniors" 2000).

The problems associated with the Canadian health care system are the result of political differences between an increasingly ideologically divided government. One outcome of such division is the potential for significant change to the health care system. As politicians battle over how best to fix the system, the people of Canada have also begun to question their health care system. Recent public opinion polls indicate a growing dissatisfaction with the Canadian health care system (Blendon et al. 1995; Donelan et al. 1999). As recently as ten years ago, Canadians were among the most satisfied in the industrialized world with their health care system (Blendon et al. 1990). What happened and why? This chapter examines the structure and problems of the Canadian health care system. As in chapter 2, I also address differential health outcomes on the basis of age, social class, sex, and race and ethnicity among Canadians. But first, let's place the Canadian system in historical perspective.

## HISTORY OF THE CANADIAN HEALTH CARE SYSTEM

The Canadian health care system has its beginnings in the treatment modalities and belief systems of the indigenous populations. By the middle of the nineteenth century, the diseases and their methods of treatment brought by immigrants were influencing Canadian health care. The professionalization of medicine began to emerge as homeopaths and eclectics were included as members of the licensing body for physicians. Also, medical schools were developed in conjunction with universities, thus limiting the proliferation of diploma mills. These efforts, although limiting the growth of the profession, improved the status of its members (Torrance 1998).

Organizationally, the Canadian health care system is grounded in the British North American Act of 1867 within which responsibility for health care was ceded to provincial governments, who "lacked the taxing power to finance large-scale health insurance programs" (Charles and Badgley 1999: 119). However, the federal government had the power to tax, but not the right to provide health care. As a result, health care was initially an individual responsibility, although some provincial governments (Ontario and Quebec) provided funding (Charles and Badgley 1999).

Historically, the province of Saskatchewan has led the movement for innovative efforts at health care reform. In 1914, a small community in Saskatchewan provided a yearly stipend of $1,500 to retain a physician. By 1916, the Rural Municipalities Act allowed communities to raise taxes for the purpose of securing the services of a physician. Depending on whether the physician worked full or part time determined the amount paid and the range of duties expected. Communities in Saskatchewan were also empowered to join together and levy taxes to pay for the construction and operation of what were referred to as union hospitals. Finally, rural communities were allowed to levy a land tax for the purpose of providing hospital insurance (Dickinson 1993).

Canada's involvement in World War I provided an impetus for change within the health care system. According to Taylor (1990), rejection rates of Canadian military recruits during World War I ranged upward to 50%. In 1919, national health insurance was proposed but not adopted. The proposal was an effort by the Liberal Party to placate the rising tide of discontent among the working class against a capitalist economic system. According to Swartz (1998), "Health insurance was as much about insuring capitalism against socialism as it was about improving workers' health, but that health insurance need not, (and in Canada did not), even imply 'nationalizing' the production and distribution of health services" (537).

Later, however, the economic devastation of the Great Depression provided fertile ground for the emergence of socialist ideals in many of the provinces, particularly in the Great Plains. For example, the League for Social Reconstruction was created in Saskatchewan in 1932. Although the league identified state health insurance as one of its main proposals, it was never enacted. By the 1940s, "public support for universal health care was strong" (Graig 1999: 124) because of the experiences associated with the Great Depression and the involvement of Canada in World War II (Taylor 1986). Connecting the impact of the depression and the development of Medicare, Armstrong and Armstrong (1996) state that,

Medicare was based on the same knowledge, the same recognition of shared vulnerability and collective responsibility. It was designed both to ensure that the bills were paid and that no particular individual would suffer economic ruin as a result of illness. (155)

Although a formal proposal was submitted to the House of Commons in 1943, action was not taken because of the political strength and diversity of the provinces (Lassey, Lassey, and Jinks 1997). Nevertheless, the first public health insurance program was established in 1946 in Swift Current, Saskatchewan (Canadian Health Coalition 2000a). This was followed in 1947 by the introduction of provincial hospital insurance in Saskatchewan (see, for example, Blakeney 1993). Throughout the 1950s, efforts to estab-

*p ¹ st pL*

lish national hospital insurance continued with passage of a national Hospital Insurance Act in 1957. In 1962, Saskatchewan was the first province to offer a public health program (Dickinson 1993). Three years later, efforts were underway for the establishment of a national health insurance program. The following year, a national Medicare program was enacted (the Medical Care Act) with the federal government agreeing to a 50-50 cost sharing of health care expenses with the provinces. Enactment of the program within the provinces and territories began the following year and was completed in April 1972 with the Yukon Territory being the last to establish its program (Canadian Health Coalition 2000a; Leatt and Williams 1997; Taylor 1990).

The foundation of the Canadian health system is built on the following principles, agreed on by the provinces and the federal government with the passage of hospital insurance in 1958 and health insurance in 1968 (see Figure 3.1). The accessibility principle was added with the passage of the Canada Health Act of 1984 (Taylor 1986).

Prior to the enactment of Medicare, health care expenditures in the United States and Canada were similar. In fact, in 1960, health care expenditures as a percentage of GDP were greater in Canada than the United States (5.4% and 5.1%, respectively). By 1970, health care expenditures as a percentage of GDP were almost identical (7.0% in Canada and 7.1% in the United States). Within ten years, significant differences were evident as health care expenditures in Canada increased only to 7.2% of GDP while the United States grew to 8.9%. The gap in health care expenditures has continued to widen, with Canada spending 9.2% of GDP on health care expenditures in 1997 compared with 13.4% for the United States (National Center for Health Statistics 2000).

Passage of the Canada Health Act of 1984 reaffirmed the basic principles on which the health system was established. Since passage of the Canada Health Act of 1984, however, the Canadian health care system

**Figure 3.1**
**Principles of the Canadian Health Care System**

- Public Administration: requires all provincial health plans to be administered and operated on a nonprofit basis.
- Comprehensiveness: requires all provincial plans to ensure that physicians and hospitals provide all medically necessary services.
- Universality: ensures that all citizens are entitled to health services and the conditions and terms of these services are uniform.
- Accessibility: requires all provincial plans to provide reasonable access to physician and hospital services. For example, extra billing for services is illegal and provincial health care plans cannot discriminate on the basis of age, sex, income, etc.
- Portability: provides coverage between provinces or when traveling outside Canada.

*Source:* Health Canada 1999: 3.

has experienced fiscal constraints. The Mulroney government in the latter 1980s and early 1990s cut the share of federal responsibility from 30.8% to 23.5%. Further cuts were made to the 1995 federal budget presented by the newly elected Liberal government. As a result, these cuts "threaten the federal government's capacity to enforce the Medicare principles" (Gray 1998: 930). Nevertheless, Canadians remain committed to the preservation of Medicare (Canadian Health Coalition 2000b). The dynamics of the Canadian health care system represent "a balancing act among federal and provincial jurisdictions along with provincial and national medical associations under the watchful scrutiny of Canadian consumers" (Leslie 1997: 68).

Efforts to undermine the public system of health care have been ongoing. For example, as the percentage of health care expenditures paid by the federal government declined, some provincial governments have attempted to limit the amount of health care by requiring an explicit definition of *medically necessary services*. Those services not so defined could then be relegated to the private sector rather than considered a public responsibility (Charles and Badgley 1999). The concept of medical necessity has evoked a number of meanings that include the following:

- What physicians and hospitals do
- The maximum we can afford
- What is scientifically justified
- What is consistently publicly funded across provinces. (Charles et al. 1997: 370)

The implications of these meanings are significant. For example, the first meaning refers to a federal floor of services, and the second implies that the same services are a provincial ceiling. The third meaning would require scientific evidence as the basis for determining services that are medically necessary, whereas the fourth meaning creates a standard package of services, regardless of location in Canada.

## FINANCING AND DELIVERY OF SERVICES

As with all health care systems, methods of financing and the delivery of services continue to evolve. The Canadian system is no exception. Currently, Canada is spending 9.2% of its GDP on health care, or approximately $2,900 per capita. Disaggregating health expenditures reveals changes over the past 20 years. In 1979, hospitals accounted for 42.5% of health expenditures. In 1999, health care expenditures for hospitals decreased to 31.6%. Similarly, health care expenditures on physicians decreased from 14.9% in 1979 to 13.9% in 1999. In contrast, health care expenditures on drugs increased from 8.6% to 15.2% between 1979 and 1999 (Canadian Institute for Health Information 2000). Canada, however, has maintained administrative costs at extremely low levels. In 1960, total expenditures on health administration and insurance was 2.7% of the total cost of health care. In 1999, only 2.3% of the total cost of health care was spent on administration and insurance (Organization for Economic Cooperation and Development 2000).

Angus (1998) identifies three historical phases of expenditures within Canadian health. The first occurred during the 1960s when health care expenditures increased because of expanding public coverage for medical and hospital services. During the 1970s, health care spending was stabilized because of wage and price controls. Finally, during the 1980s, health care expenditures again increased. Examining the distribution of health care expenditures, Angus (1998) argues that increases throughout the 1980s occurred primarily within the institutional sector, particularly long-term care facilities. Because of shifting demographics throughout the industrialized world, the Canadian experience is not unique. If the nations of the developed world expect to control the overall cost of health care, they must address how they will finance their long-term care needs. Although significant, long-term care needs represents only one, albeit increasingly important, component of the health care system.

The two most significant legislative reforms since the passage of Medicare are the Established Programs Financing Act of 1977 (EPF) and the Canada Health Act of 1984. These two measures fundamentally altered the economic relationship between the federal and provincial governments relative to Medicare. Since their inception, provincial governments have had increasing power over the definition and provision of Medicare. At the same time, the role of the federal government has diminished.

Implementation of the Established Programs Financing Act of 1977 (EPF) fundamentally altered the relationship between the national and provincial governments regarding health care. Passage of this legislation meant that federal monies that had been in the form of cost sharing with provinces were now block grants determined by the rate of growth in the GDP. As a result, "the federal government effectively shifted the responsibility to exercise restraint over health care costs to the provinces" (Maioni 1998: 173). The long-term outcome has been a significant increase in the cost of health care to the provinces. When Medicare was initially developed, the cost of health care was split evenly between the federal and provincial governments. In 1980, the federal government contributed approximately one-third the cost of health care. By the 1990s, the federal contribution to provincial health care had diminished to less than 25%. The shift in financial responsibility for health care gave provincial governments greater control over the prioritization of health care services. Similarly, the federal government had greater stability regarding health expenditures. The introduction of block grants by the federal government also ensured equality in per capita health expenditures between the provinces (Taylor 1990). Introduction of the EPF also led to a "balkaniza- tion of provincial health insurance plans, some of which began to levy higher plan 'premiums' on residents, while others allowed physicians to 'extra-bill' for services above those insured under Medicare" (Leatt and Williams 1997: 4). This led to the second major reform, the Canada Health Act of 1984.

One of the most significant pieces of health legislation in Canadian his- tory, the Canada Health Act fundamentally altered the relationship between physicians and patients (you can download an overview of the act at www.hc-sc.gc.ca/medicare/chaover.html). The Canada Health Act "defined more precisely the conditions upon which federal payments would continue" (Taylor 1990: 169). Specifically, provinces were required to "provide reasonable compensation for *all* medically necessary insured services" (Taylor 1990: 170). In addition, the act stipulated the quid pro quo withholding of payments to provinces if they allowed extra billing. Although extra billing had been defended as an issue of maintaining qual- ity and control, Globerman (1990) argues that "economic interests and antiwelfare views bolstered the professional defense of extra-billing as needed to protect the quality of health care" (22). The response of provinces to the act varied. British Columbia had outlawed the practice prior to the act, whereas the provincial government of Alberta supported the right of physicians to extra bill (Taylor 1990). By 1987, however, extra billing in all provinces was nonexistent (Organization for Economic Coop- eration and Development 1994).

Because of a sagging economy in the latter 1980s and early 1990s, the Canadian government passed the Expenditures Restraint Act. Its purpose was to place a cap on federal health expenditures to provincial govern- ments (Leatt and Williams 1997). This effort, as well as previous legislative attempts to control health care spending, has had a disastrous effect on the Canadian health care system. In particular, as health care costs have increased, provinces have had to limit the availability of services by clos- ing hospitals. Because the provincial health care systems rely on tax rev- enues for their health care system, any slowdown in their economy will have a similar impact on their revenue stream for health care services. Health care in Canada is financed primarily through "provincial tax rev- enues and federal government transfers" (Eyles, Birch, and Newbold 1995: 324). More specifically, these revenues are identified as "province- specific taxes within the national income tax program, and...equalization payments designed to smooth out the interprovincial differences in aver- age per capita income" (Naylor 1999: 12).

Provincial governments have experienced continued reductions in fed- eral funding as well as increased political conservatism. In 1994, the EPF and the Canada Assistance Plan "were replaced with a new Canada

Health and Social Transfer (CHST), a large block grant, with no conditions other than the five Medicare principles" (Gray 1998: 930). The steadily decreasing economic role of the federal government reduces its ability to enforce the five principles on which Medicare is premised. As a result, the future of the Canadian health care system lies in one of two possible directions.

The conservative approach would allow provinces the opportunity to create a two-tiered American-style health care system. Examples of privatization include the removal of services once covered by Medicare; shifting covered services out of Medicare; and "contracting out of 'non-core' medical services (labs, ambulances and rehab services) to private companies" (Canadian Health Coalition 2000b: 2). In the province of Alberta, the premier has proposed constructing private hospitals to reduce the waiting period for surgery. Allan Rock, the Canadian minister of health, argues that public hospitals in Alberta already exist but are not performing surgeries because of the lack of funds (Iglehart 2000b).

Alternatively, the future of Canadian health care lies in keeping with the philosophy of health care as a social good. Canada could return to its roots and reestablish Medicare in its original framework. Historically, Medicare has made Canadians one of the most satisfied populations with their health care system in the industrialized world (Charles and Badgley, 1999). Interestingly, one of the major arguments against Medicare has been the presumed increased reliance by Canadians on the American health care system. Although anecdotal evidence of Canadians utilizing American hospitals because of shortages and long waiting lists in Canada exist, Katz, Verrilli, and Barer (1998) report that such outcomes have little basis in reality. Examining out-of-country spending by the Ontario Health Insurance Plan, Katz et al. (1998) argue that health expenditures in the United States are primarily the result of two conditions. First, some Canadians spend significant amounts of time in the United States during the winter months (so-called snowbirds) and need emergency medical services. Second are those Canadians who are seeking specific health care that is generally more available in the United States than Canada. It is also important to remember that Americans travel to Canada for services as well (for example, less expensive prescription drugs).

### Physicians

As Armstrong and Armstrong (1998) point out, the payment method for physician services continues to be debated. Throughout the development of national health insurance in Canada, the role of the physician has been a contentious issue. When Saskatchewan inaugurated provincial health care in 1962, physicians in the province went on strike. Physicians also opposed movement toward a nationwide health insurance system in the early 1970s and continue to take political action (see Sibbald 1998). However, Williams et al. (1995) suggest that physicians in Canada are becoming less ideological and more pragmatic in their acceptance of Medicare. As Coburn (1993) documents, physicians in Canada are experiencing a decline in medical dominance. This decline represents the changing dynamics associated within 12 health care systems also experiencing change as a result of political and economic uncertainty.

Currently, provincial medical associations negotiate with provincial governments regarding fees for physicians (Coburn 1993) who are primarily engaged in private practice throughout the country. Although these negotiations determine the percentage increase over the previous fee schedule, "medical associations are generally free to reallocate spending among general practitioners and specialists" (Organization for Economic Cooperation and Development 1994: 107). Global budgeting gives provincial governments an economic framework within which to constrain health care costs. The application of global budgeting is not unique to the Canadian system because most Western industrialized nations utilize it in some format (Lassey et al. 1997).

Canadians are free to choose their physician, but access to most specialists and admission to a hospital is generally through their general/family practitioner. Although Canadian physicians provide services on a fee-for-service basis, patients do not receive a bill. Rather, physicians bill the province for the services they perform and are reimbursed on the basis of the negotiated fee schedule. Some specialists get around provincial fee schedules by charging for services "not expressly described in the benefits schedule (for example, telephone consultations, letter for employers, photocopying of records, or even, in the extreme, booking operating room time)" (Naylor 1999: 18). There is increasing interest to change the physician reimbursement method from fee for service to capitation. In other words, physicians would have a roster of patients and receive an agreed-upon amount per patient, regardless of the number of visits per year.

Throughout the 1970s and 1980s, the number of physicians in Canada was increasing at a rate faster than the general population. More recently, their rate of growth has been slowing (Lassey et al. 1997) "although not because of a lack of applicants" (Reamy 1991: 217). According to the Canadian Medical Association, the number of graduates from Canadian medical schools peaked in 1974 at 2,650. By 1997, Canadian medical schools graduated 1,822 doctors (Canadian Medical Association 2001). Furthermore, "The federal government, by agreement with the provinces, has attempted to limit overall supply by placing restrictions on the immigration of foreign physicians" (Burke and Stevenson 1998: 606). According to the Canadian Medical Association (2001), the number of immigrants to Canada who identified medicine as their occupation has decreased from a high of 1,347 in 1969 to 245 in 1997.

The outcome of these efforts is a potential physician shortage (Evans 1998) as evidenced by the 2% decline from 187 physicians per 100,000 in 1989 to 183 per 100,000 in 1997 (Canadian Institute for Health Information 2000). General practitioners and specialists, as a percentage of total health employment, also decreased throughout the 1990s. In 1990, general practitioners constituted 4.1% of total health employment. By 1994, general practitioners were 3.9% of total health employment. Specialists constituted 3.7% and 3.6%, respectively. The density of general practitioners and specialists per 1,000 population remained steady throughout the 1990s at 0.9%. On a more positive note, 23.6% of all physicians in Canada were female in 1990. By 1998, the percentage of physicians who were female increased to 29.5% (Organization for Economic Cooperation and Development 2000).

## Hospitals

Hospitals in Canada are generally private, nonprofit institutions "owned by voluntary organizations, municipal/provincial authorities, and to a decreasing degree by religious orders" (Organization for Economic Cooperation and Development 1994: 105). For-profit health care facilities generally provide long-term care or specialized services (Health Canada 1999). According to the Canada Health Act, "health care in hospitals involves much more than treatment and cure. The Act specifically names those things deemed necessary for health care" (Armstrong and Armstrong 1998: 63). These include the following:

- Basic needs such as meals and a room
- Diagnosis and tests that are determined to be medically necessary
- Treatment determined to be medically necessary
- Supplies and equipment necessary while in the hospital
- Drugs and other preparations given as part of the hospital regimen to treat the patient
- Health care providers necessary for the diagnosis and treatment of the patient. (Armstrong and Armstrong 1998)

As in most industrialized nations, the largest share of health care costs is hospital related. As a result, hospitals have borne the brunt of provincial health care cuts (Roos et al. 1998). According to Iglehart (2000a), the number of acute care hospitals and beds decreased significantly between 1991 and 1999. The Organization for Economic Cooperation and Development (2000) reports total in-patient care beds per 1,000 decreased from 6.3 in 1990 to 4.7 in 1997. Similarly, the average length of stay, which had increased from 11.1 in 1960 to 13.1 in 1980, had decreased to 8.4 in 1997, and the average number of acute care staff per bed peaked in 1990 at 2.80 (Organization for Economic Cooperation and Development 2000). Roos et al. (1998) argue that the decrease in hospital beds in Winnipeg, Manitoba, has not affected the overall delivery of care to those most in need. Furthermore, with regard to access to surgery, Roos et al. (1998) report that "access to high-profile surgical procedures actually increased during the five-year period" (241). Given the continued efforts to cut health care costs, particularly within the hospital sector, outcomes do not appear to be affected. For example, a recent examination of survival from 15 forms of cancer among low-income patients in Detroit, Michigan, and Toronto, Ontario, found "a significant Toronto survival advantage for 13 of 15 cancer sites" (Gorey et al. 1997: 1160). The authors conclude that these differences are best explained as a result of differences in health care systems.

As with physicians, provincial governments negotiate with hospitals regarding their budgets. As a result, provinces exercise considerable control over the delivery of hospital services. For example, "in Ontario, hospitals receive a base budget, an inflation increase, and a growth funding component to compensate for increased volume" (Reamy 1991: 214). In addition, hospital operating and capital spending budgets are separate, providing provincial governments control over the addition of new hospital services or technology. As White (1995) points out, provinces may cover only a portion of the cost for capital expenses, requiring hospitals to raise the remainder through private sources. Global budgeting of hospitals can create problems of inefficiency, particularly as the patient mix changes. As a result, provinces are experimenting with a new form of hospital funding based on patient mix (Fooks 1999). Regardless, one of the most dramatic differences between hospitals in Canada and the United States is in terms of administrative costs. Because of a single-payer system providing the primary source of hospital financing, paperwork is limited and so is the necessary staff.

## CURRENT REALITIES AND THE ROLE OF THE STATE

The current realities associated with the Canadian health care system are inextricably interconnected to the role of the state. It is within this context that this section addresses why Medicare is facing the most serious challenge to its fundamental principles and ultimate existence.

According to Armstrong and Armstrong (1998), the problems with the Canadian health care system include an increasing reliance on prescription drugs, fee-for-service payments, and privatization. Prescription drug prices increased dramatically in the last two decades of the twentieth century. Armstrong and Armstrong (1998) argue that drug prices have increased for three reasons. First, most provinces have not established universal drug plans. Second, compulsory licensing "allowed the importing, manufacture, sale, and use of generic copies of the brand-name drugs before their patents expired" (134). Third, there has been a greater emphasis on treatment regimens utilizing expensive new drug therapies.

Armstrong and Armstrong (1998) also identify fee-for-service (FFS) as a problem area because it contributes to the overall cost of health care in Canada. Instead, they suggest movement toward a system in which physicians are salaried.

Finally, they point to efforts at privatization as a problem for the Canadian health care system. Using the United States as an example, they question how privatizing health services will maintain the five principles on which the Canadian health care system was built. Indeed, they suggest "these problems are arising as a consequence of strategies for reform, or a move to a more private, multi-payer approach to heath care" (Armstrong and Armstrong 1998: 142). Currently, supplementary benefits differ between provinces. Buske (1998) identifies differences among provinces regarding coverage of health care benefits such as vision, dental, and prescription drugs. Although in-hospital prescription drugs are covered for all residents in all provinces, out-of-hospital drug programs vary by province. According to Freund et al. (2000), each province determines its policy regarding access, coverage, and co-payments for prescription drugs. Some provinces provide universal drug coverage; others offer private coverage for drugs.

Perhaps the most controversial reform effort is the current effort to regionalize health services. According to Lomas, Woods, and Veenstra (1997), decision-making power has been devolved in all but one province (Ontario). Although the regionalization boards cannot raise revenue, they "are responsible for local planning, setting priorities, allocating funds and managing services for greater effectiveness and efficiency, within provincially defined broad core services" (Lomas et al. 1997: 373). Furthermore, board members must satisfy three competing constituencies: the provincial government, the providers, and the community members (Lomas, Veenstra, and Woods 1997).

The process of regionalization involves a realignment (upward as well as downward) of authority and responsibility with an expected outcome of greater efficiency and reduced cost. Although regionalization differs among provinces, Church and Barker (1998) identify five characteristics of the process that transcend political boundaries. First is the development of an organizational board composed of either appointed or elected officials. For example, the regionalization board in Saskatchewan replaced some four hundred boards that had represented hospitals, nursing homes, and other health-related functions within the province. Second, most regionalization boards engage in some form of global budgeting. Third, is the shifting of service delivery from an institutional to community-based settings. Fourth, is a change in how programs are assessed. In other words,

**Figure 3.2**
**Future Concerns**

| |
|---|
| • Broadening the definition of health |
| • Promoting health and preventing disease |
| • Community-based care |
| • Increased participation |
| • Regional authorities |
| • Human resource planning |
| • Provincial planning and coordination |
| • Research |
| • Other recommendations |

*Source:* Mhatre and Derber 1998.

regionalization boards would assess outcomes of services rather than inputs. Fifth, is the reduction in the size of provincial departments of health (Church and Barker 1998). Although most provinces have adopted some form of regionalization, there is no guarantee that the desired outcomes will be realized. And, as Lomas (1997) points out, "it is difficult to generalize about the performance of 123 devolved authorities in 9 provinces" (822).

Finally, the role of provincial governments relative to the Canadian health care system can be understood in the various health policy themes that have been developed. These themes reflect future concerns for Medicare and are presented in Figure 3.2.

These themes provide provinces with a framework for continued analysis of their individual systems. For example, Mhatre and Derber (1998) point to the implications of a broader definition of health. All Canadians are guaranteed equal access to health care, but there are concerns regarding equity of services received. As provinces expand the meaning of health to include not only the physical, but also the social and economic environments, the health of Canadians may be questioned as problems of water and air pollution or inadequate housing are factored into the definition of health. Although these themes raise future concerns, health differences already exist among Canadians and are examined in the following section.

## THE HEALTH OF THE POPULATION BY AGE, SEX, SOCIAL CLASS, AND RACE AND ETHNICITY

Although the Canadian system of health care ensures all citizens access to medically necessary services, differential health outcomes based on age, sex, social class, and racial and ethnic background persist. For example, data in Table 3.1 illustrate differences in health status by age, sex, and social class.

**Table 3.1**
**Self-Rated Health Status, by Age and Sex, by Income Adequacy (Age-Standardized), and by Province, Age 12+. Canada, 1996–1997**

|  | % Excellent | % Very Good | % Good | % Fair | % Poor |
|---|---|---|---|---|---|
| Total, age 12+ | 25 | 38 | 27 | 7 | 2 |
| Male | 26 | 39 | 26 | 7 | 2 |
| Female | 24 | 38 | 27 | 8 | 2 |
| Age 12-14 Total | 32 | 41 | 25 | 2 | # |
| Male | 37 | 39 | 22 | 2 | # |
| Female | 26 | 43 | 27 | 3 | # |
| Age 15-17 Total | 29 | 43 | 23 | 4 | # |
| Male | 36 | 41 | 20 | 3 | # |
| Female | 20 | 45 | 27 | 6 | # |
| Age 18-19 Total | 25 | 50 | 22 | 3 | # |
| Male | 29 | 51 | 17 | 3 | # |
| Female | 22 | 49 | 26 | 3 | # |
| Age 20-24 Total | 34 | 40 | 22 | 3 | 0 |
| Male | 38 | 37 | 21 | 3 | # |
| Female | 30 | 43 | 24 | 3 | # |
| Age 25–34 Total | 31 | 42 | 22 | 4 | 1 |
| Male | 30 | 44 | 21 | 4 | 1 |
| Female | 31 | 41 | 23 | 5 | 1 |
| Age 35-44 Total | 26 | 41 | 26 | 5 | 1 |
| Male | 26 | 42 | 26 | 5 | 1 |
| Female | 27 | 40 | 26 | 5 | 1 |
| Age 45-54 Total | 24 | 38 | 27 | 8 | 2 |
| Male | 25 | 39 | 26 | 7 | 2 |
| Female | 23 | 38 | 27 | 9 | 2 |
| Age 55-64 Total | 19 | 33 | 32 | 12 | 5 |
| Male | 20 | 32 | 31 | 12 | 5 |
| Female | 18 | 34 | 31 | 12 | 5 |
| Age 65-74 Total | 13 | 29 | 38 | 15 | 5 |
| Male | 14 | 30 | 34 | 17 | 6 |
| Female | 13 | 28 | 41 | 13 | 4 |
| Age 75+ Total | 10 | 26 | 37 | 19 | 8 |
| Male | 9 | 26 | 39 | 17 | 8 |
| Female | 11 | 26 | 35 | 21 | 7 |
|  |  |  |  |  |  |
| Lowest Income | 19 | 28 | 32 | 16 | 5 |
| Lower Middle Income | 18 | 32 | 32 | 14 | 5 |
| Middle Income | 22 | 39 | 29 | 8 | 2 |
| Upper Middle Income | 26 | 41 | 26 | 6 | 1 |
| Highest Income | 33 | 40 | 22 | 4 | 1 |
| Income not stated | 27 | 37 | 27 | 8 | 3 |

These differences remain because of differential opportunities in the environmental, physical, and economic environments within which people live, and they will continue to shape the landscape of Canada. Also, as noted earlier, differences also exist among provinces regarding the coverage of services such as vision and dental care.

**Table 3.1 (continued)**

| | | | | | |
|---|---|---|---|---|---|
| Newfoundland | 26 | 45 | 20 | 7 | # |
| Prince Edward Island | 22 | 45 | 23 | 8 | # |
| Nova Scotia | 20 | 43 | 25 | 10 | # |
| New Brunswick | 21 | 37 | 31 | 9 | # |
| Quebec | 27 | 37 | 28 | 1 | 1 |
| Ontario | 25 | 39 | 25 | 7 | 3 |
| Manitoba | 21 | 39 | 29 | 8 | 2 |
| Saskatchewan | 17 | 39 | 34 | 8 | # |
| Alberta | 25 | 38 | 26 | 7 | 2 |
| British Columbia | 25 | 38 | 29 | 7 | 2 |

# Data suppressed because of high sampling variability.

*Source:* Statistics Canada, *National Population Health Survey, 1996–97,* Special tabulations.

*Source:* Statistics Canada, Catalogue Number H39-467/1999E, *Statistical Report on the Health of Canadians,* 1999. Table 53, Self-rated health status, by age and sex, by income adequacy (age-standardized) and by province, age 12+, Canada, 1996–97, p. 219.

*Source:* Self-rated health status, by age and sex, by income adequacy (age-standardized) and by province, age 12+, Canada, 1996-97. From the Statistics Canada publication, "Statistical Report on the Health of Canadians." Catalogue No. 82-570, 1999, page 219.

Statistics Canada information is used with the permission of the Minister of Industry, as Minister responsible for Statistics Canada. Information on the availability of the wide range of data from Statistics Canada can be obtained from Statistics Canada's Regional Offices, its World Wide Web site at http://www.statcan.ca, and its toll-free number: 1-800-263-1136.

## Age

As an industrialized nation, Canada is also experiencing a demographic shift of its population. Although relatively young by comparison, the population aged 65 and over will continue to increase in the twenty-first century. According to the U.S. Bureau of the Census (1992), the aging population in Canada will increase from 11.5% of the population in 1990 to 14.3% in 2010 and 20.7% in 2025. More importantly, the oldest-old population will more than double, from 2.4% to 5.2% between 1990 and 2025.

In general, the health status of the aging population in Canada is consistent with other industrialized nations. That is, Canadians over the age of 65 are less likely to report their health status as excellent and more likely to identify it as fair or poor (Statistics Canada 1999). Furthermore, the percentage of Canadian elderly with low income has been increasing. In 1980, just over one-third of the elderly experienced low incomes. By the early 1990s, this had declined to 19% in 1994–1995, but increased to 21% in 1996 (Statistics Canada 1999).

The growth in the aging population is expected to strain the Canadian health care system as demand for services increases. This is particularly evident with regard to hospital and long-term care needs (Lassey et al.

1997). For example, the *Statistical Report on the Health of Canadians* (Statistics Canada 1999) reports that the average length of stay in 1995–1996 among those aged 65 to 74 was 14 days. Among those aged 75 and over, the average length of stay was 23 days. By comparison, the average length of stay for all ages was 11 days. Furthermore, Canadian elderly, who are 12% of the population, account "for 31 percent of acute hospital stays and half of the days in hospitals" (Canadian Institute for Health Information 2000: 41). The most recent estimates indicate that in 1994, 40% of total health care spending in Canada was on the elderly (Anderson and Hussey 2000). By comparison, 38% of total health care spending in the United States in 1995 was on the elderly. However, per capita health care spending on the elderly in 1997 was $6,764 in Canada and $12,090 in the United States (Anderson and Hussey 2000). Canadian elderly, in comparison with aging populations in other industrialized nations, are among the most satisfied with their health care system. The elderly in Canada are also less likely to experience problems paying for the health care they need (Donelan et al. 2000).

The demographic shift toward an older population is a reality in Canada, but increased health care costs are not necessarily an inevitable consequence. Evans (1987) argues that these demographic changes will have little economic impact on the ability of the Canadian health care system's ability to provide services. According to Evans (1987) "the increases in health care costs…will be supportable by the allocation of a constant, or even falling, share of our national income" (167).

### Sex

As with other industrialized countries, health outcomes in Canada differ between males and females. According to the World Health Organization (2000), Canada has one of the highest life expectancy rates in the world. The most recent data place life expectancy at birth for males at 76.2 years and 81.9 for females. These differences persist regardless of the province or territory (Statistics Canada 1999).

In addition to life expectancy differences, differences in health problems and outcomes exist between males and females in Canada. For example, according to the *Statistical Report on the Health of Canadians* (Statistics Canada 1999), females experience higher prevalence rates for chronic conditions such as food and nonfood allergies, arthritis/rheumatism, back problems, high blood pressure, migraine headaches, and asthma. New cases and deaths due to cancer, however, are higher among males. In addition, males experience higher mortality rates for all major causes of death.

Hospitalization rates differ between males and females depending on the cause. For example, women experience higher hospitalization rates for cancer, whereas men are more likely to be hospitalized for respiratory and circulatory problems (Statistics Canada 1999). Women are also more likely than men are to visit a physician. Given these variations in health, males, regardless of age, are more likely to report their health status as excellent or good (D'Arcy 1998a).

## Social Class

Although Canada has a health care system that ensures universal access, class-related health outcomes persist in Canada. According to the *Canadian National Forum Report* (1997), "the wealthiest Canadians can expect to live four years longer than the poorest Canadians" (n.p.). Furthermore, Health Canada (2000) concludes that such differences remain regardless of age, sex, race, or place of residence (see also Badgley 1991; Frohlich and Mustard 1996). According to the data from Health Canada, wealthier Canadians are more likely to identify their health status as excellent or good when compared with economically poorer Canadians.

In an extensive analysis of the relationship between social class and health-related outcomes, D'Arcy (1998b) argues that lower class Canadians experience higher rates of morbidity and mortality. For example, in 1986, the infant mortality rate among lower income Canadians was 11 per 1,000 live births, whereas it was almost 50% lower (6 per 1,000 live births) for higher income Canadians. According to D'Arcy (1998b), "infants in the lowest income quintile are 83 percent more likely to die than those in the highest income quintile" (81).

Similarly, although life expectancy rates for males and females by income level have diminished, differences remain. D'Arcy (1998b) also reports that although health behaviors and outcomes by income levels are decreasing, differences in the likelihood of death, disability, risk behaviors, preventive health practices, and utilization of services and well-being remain. He argues that further reduction in health differences by social class will require economic changes such as lowering wage differentials and improved benefit packages for all employees. Further evidence of class-based differences with regard to health is reflected in the percentage of Canadians with supplemental dental, corrective eyewear, and prescription drug coverage. The data in Table 3.2 illustrate differences in supplemental insurance rates by social class. Without access to supplemental insurance, poorer Canadians are less likely to have access to those therapeutic regimens that could provide improved health status or increase life expectancy.

Health outcome differences are not confined to a comparison between the richest and poorest residents of Canada. In Winnipeg, Manitoba, "the health of residents in middle income neighborhoods is poor compared with that of people living in higher income neighborhoods" (Roos and Mustard 1997: 101).

**Table 3.2**
**The Great Divide: Insurance by Education and Income**
**Percentage of Canadians by Education and Income Who Reported Some**
**Insurance Coverage, 1998–1999**

|  | Dental Care | Corrective Eyewear | Prescription Drugs |
|---|---|---|---|
| **Level of Education** | | | |
| Less than H.S. | 48% | 45% | 71% |
| High School | 55% | 52% | 72% |
| College | 59% | 51% | 75% |
| University | 66% | 60% | 80% |
| **Level of Income** | | | |
| Lowest Income | 30% | 29% | 58% |
| Lower Middle | 41% | 37% | 66% |
| Upper Middle | 65% | 59% | 80% |
| Highest Income | 79% | 70% | 87% |
| Not Stated | 50% | 46% | 73% |

*Source:* © 2000, CIHI., Table 18, p. 21, "The Great Divide: Insurance by Education and Income who reported some insurance coverage in 1998/99." In *Health Care in Canada: A First Annual Report*, copied with permission. Published by the Canadian Institute for Health Information, Ottawa, Canada.

### Race and Ethnicity

Although Canada is considerably more racially and ethnically homogeneous than the United States, health outcomes are generally poorer for the indigenous population. According to D'Arcy (1998b), "native Indian and Inuit populations have significantly poorer health and much shorter life expectancy than the rest of Canadians" (74). These differences have remained, and, in some cases, increased. According to the *Canadian National Forum on Health* (1997), there is a seven-year difference in life expectancy between the aboriginal and nonaboriginal populations. Furthermore, the aboriginal population is twice as likely to be in poverty compared with the Canadian-born population. As a result, delivery of health care to native populations is of concern to health professionals (Lassey et al. 1997).

The health of recent immigrants is generally comparable to Canadian-born citizens. In particular, non-European immigrants, regardless of sex, have longer life expectancies (D'Arcy 1998b). According to the *Statistical Report on the Health of Canadians* (Statistics Canada 1999), immigrants are primarily from European countries, the United States, Hong Kong, India, or China.

### CONCLUSION

The Canadian health care system, like all systems in the industrialized world, is undergoing change. The Canadian system, commonly referred to as Medicare, evolved over decades of provincial experimentation, debate, and negotiation. By law, health care is a provincial responsibility. Thus, in reality, the Canadian health care system is a patchwork of ten provincial and two territorial systems, and it is more accurately described as socialized insurance rather than socialized medicine. Initially, the federal government provided matching (50-50) funding to provincial governments for health care. That percentage has dropped below 25% today, but efforts are underway to increase the federal participation levels—an effort to stave off provincial threats to undermine the basic principles on which Medicare was founded, which include universality, public administration, comprehensiveness, portability, and accessibility (added as a result of the Canadian Health Act of 1984).

Although the system offers universal access and portability, health outcome differences among population groups exist, particularly on the basis of social class position. Nevertheless, the Canadian health care system offers considerable evidence that a multigovernment partnership can effectively create and manage health care for its citizens. In its effort not to create a two-tiered system, the Canadian system remains unique in its opposition to a parallel private system available to its wealthier citizens. The system does, however, allow citizens to purchase private insurance to cover costs not borne by the provincial systems. It is this role of the state, relative to health access and outcomes, that separates the Canadian system from other industrialized nations.

Although the Canadian health care system is unarguably experiencing a crisis of confidence, it remains strongly committed to maintaining the principles on which it was founded. Future changes in the system appear to be more focused on the delivery of care and methods of payment rather than changing the financing mechanism. For example, Allen Rock, the current minister of health, suggests changes in the delivery of primary health care that would allow patient access to a defined group of health care professionals rather than utilizing emergency rooms. In addition, Rock argues for changing the physician compensation from a fee for service to capitation (Iglehart 2000b).

Finally, the Canadian health care system must address the economic and social ramifications associated with an increasingly older population. Given the history of the Canadian health care system, it is expected to create a health policy that will ensure the integrity and viability of this population without compromising access to medically necessary medications and treatment regimens. Armstrong and Armstrong (1996) are less optimistic as they warn of "increasing inequality, fewer choices, and less skilled care" (226). Thus the Canadian health care system of national health insurance will persist, but with alterations. These changes "have to do with the goals, shape, pace and political character of the Canadian reform initiative" (Adams 1994: 141). The early twenty-first century will be a defining period for the Canadian health care system.

## REFERENCES

Adams, N. Duane. 1994. "The Future and Long-Range Planning of Health Care Services: Canada." In *Health Care Systems in Canada & the United Kingdom: Can They Deliver?* ed. Kenneth Lee. Keele, UK: Ryburn Publishing.

Anderson, Gerard F., and Peter Sotir Hussey. 2000. "Population Aging: A Comparison among Industrialized Countries." *Health Affairs* 19(3): 191–203.

Andrain, Charles F. 1998. *Public Health Policies and Social Inequality.* New York: New York University Press.

Angus, Douglas E. 1998. "Health Care Costs: Canada in Perspective." In *Health and Canadian Society: Sociological Perspective,* 3rd ed., ed. David Coburn, Carl D'Arcy, and George Torrance. Toronto: University of Toronto Press.

Armstrong, Pat, and Hugh Armstrong. 1996. *Wasting Away: The Undermining of Canadian Health Care.* Toronto: Oxford University Press.

———. 1998. *Universal Health Care: What the United States Can Learn from the Canadian Experience.* New York: The New Press.

Badgley, Robin F. 1991. "Social and Economic Disparities under Canadian Health Care." *International Journal of Health Services* 21(4): 659–671.

Blakeney, Allen E. 1993. "The Political Perspective: Planning and Implementing the Canadian System." In *Looking North for Health: What We Can Learn from Canada's Health Care System,* ed. Arnold Bennett and Orvall Adams. San Francisco: Jossey-Bass.

Blendon, Robert J., Robert Leitman, Ian Morrison, and Karen Donelan. 1990. "Satisfaction with Health Systems in Ten Nations." *Health Affairs* 9(2): 185–192.

Blendon, Robert J., John Benson, Karen Donelan, Robert Leitman, Humphrey Taylor, Christen Koeck, and Daniel Gifferman. 1995. "Who Has the Best Health Care System? A Second Look." *Health Affairs* 14(4): 220–230.

Burke, M., and H. Michael Stevenson. 1998. "Fiscal Crisis and Restructuring in Medicare: The Realities of Health in Canada." In *Health and Canadian Society: Sociological Perspectives,* 3rd ed., ed. David Coburn, Carl D'Arcy, and George Torrance. Toronto: University of Toronto Press.

Buske, Lynda. 1998. "What's Covered? What's Not." *Canadian Medical Association Journal* 159(1): 120.

Canadian Health Coalition. 2000a. "A Brief History of Canada's Public Health Care." www.healthcoalition.ca/dates.html. August 22, 2000.

———. 2000b. "The Corporate Threat to Canada's Health Care System. www.healthcoalition.ca/privatization.html. August 22, 2000.

Canadian Institute for Health Information. 2000. *Health Care in Canada: A First Annual Report.* Ottawa, Ontario.

Canadian Medical Association. 2001. "Advocacy & Communications: Physician Workforce." Table II. Landed Immigrants Indicating Medicine as Their Intended Occupation and Graduates of Canadian Medical School 1967–1997. www.cma.ca/advocacy/taskforce/table2.html. January 10, 2001.

Canadian National Forum on Health. 1997. Vol. 1: *Building on the Legacy—The Final Report*. http://www.hc.ca.whatnew.htm. August 25, 1998.

Charles, Catherine A., and Robin F. Badgley. 1999. "Canadian National Health Insurance." In *Health Care Systems in Transition: An International Perspective*, ed. Francis D. Powell and Albert F. Wessen. Thousand Oaks, CA: Sage.

Charles, Cathy, Jonathan Lomas, Vandna Bhatia, and Victoria A. Vincent. 1997. "Medical Necessity in Canadian Health Policy: Four Meanings and...a Funeral?" *Milbank Quarterly* 75(3): 365–394.

Chollet, Deborah J. 1993. "Health Care Financing in Selected Industrialized Nations: Comparative Analysis and Comment." In *Trends in Health Benefits*. U.S. Department of Labor. Pension and Welfare Benefits Administration. Washington, DC: Government Printing Office.

Church, John, and Paul Barker. 1998. "Regionalization of Health Services in Canada: A Critical Perspective." *International Journal of Health Services* 28(3): 467–486.

Coburn, David. 1993. "Professional Powers in Decline: Medicine in a Changing Canada." In *The Changing Medical Profession: An International Perspective*, ed. Frederic W. Hafferty and John B. McKinlay. New York: Oxford.

Colvin, Phyllis. 1994. "Canadian Health Care Financing." In *Health Care Systems in Canada & the United Kingdom*, ed. Kenneth Lee. Keele, UK: Ryburn Publishing.

D'Arcy, Carl. 1998a. "Health Status of Canadians." In *Health and Canadian Society: Sociological Perspectives*, 3rd ed., ed. David Coburn, Carl D'Arcy, and George Torrance. Toronto: University of Toronto Press.

———. 1998b. "Social Distribution of Health among Canadians." In *Health And Canadian Society: Sociological Perspectives*, 3rd ed., ed. David Coburn, Carl D'Arcy, and George Torrance. Toronto: University of Toronto Press.

Dickinson, Harley D. 1993. "The Struggle for State Health Insurance: Reconsidering the Role of Saskatchewan Farmers." *Studies in Political Economy* 41: 133–156.

Donelan, Karen, et al. 1999. "The Cost of Health System Change: Public Discontent in Five Nations." *Health Affairs* 18(3): 206–216.

———., et al. 2000. "The Elderly in Five Nations: The Importance of Universal Coverage." *Health Affairs* 19(3): 226–235.

Evans, Robert G. 1987. "Hang Together, or Hang Separately: The Viability of a Universal Health Care System in an Aging Society." *Canadian Public Policy* 12(2): 165–180.

———. 1993. "Health Care in the Canadian Community." In *Looking North for Health: What We Can Learn from Canada's Health Care System*, ed. Arnold Bennett and Orvil Adams. San Francisco: Jossey-Bass.

———. 1998. "New Bottles, Same Old Wine: Right and Wrong on Physician Supply." *Canadian Medical Association Journal* 158(6): 757–759.

Eyles, John, Stephen Birch, and K. Bruce Newbold. 1995. "Delivering the Goods? Access to Family Physician Services in Canada: A Comparison of 1985 and 1991." *Journal of Health and Social Behavior* 36(4): 322–332.

Fooks, Catherine. 1999. "Will Power, Cost Control, and Health Reform in Canada, 1987–1992." In *Health Care Systems in Transition: An International Perspective*. ed. Frances D. Powell and Albert F. Wessen. Thousand Oaks, CA: Sage.

Freund, Deborah, et al. 2000. "Outpatient Pharmaceuticals and the Elderly: Policies in Seven Nations." *Health Affairs* 19(3): 259–266.

Frohlich, Norman, and Cam Mustard. 1996. "A Regional Comparison of Socioeconomic and Health Indices in a Canadian Province." *Social Science and Medicine* 42(9): 1273–1281.

Globerman, Judith. 1990. "Free Enterprise, Professional Ideology, and Self-Interest: An Analysis of Resistance by Canadian Physicians to Universal Health Insurance." *Journal of Health and Social Behavior* 31(1): 11–27.

Gorey, K. M., E. J. Holowary, G. Fehringer, E. Laukkamen, A. Moskowitz, D. J. Webster, and N. C. Richter. 1997. "An International Comparison of Cancer Survival: Toronto, Ontario, and Detroit, Michigan, Metropolitan Areas." *American Journal of Public Health* 87(7): 1156–1163.

Graig, Laurene A. 1999. *Health of Nations: An International Perspective on U.S. Health Care Reform.* Washington, DC: Congressional Quarterly.

Gray, Gwen. 1998. "Access to Medical Care under Strain: New Pressures in Canada and Australia." *Journal of Health Politics, Policy and Law* 23(6): 905–947.

Health Canada. 1999. "Canada's Health Care System." www.hc-sc.gc.ca/datapcb/datahesa/E-sys.html. August 23, 2000.

———. 2000. "What Makes Canadians Healthy or Unhealthy?" www.hc.sc.gc.ca/httb/phdd/determinants/e_determinants.html. August 23, 2000.

"How Many Canadian Seniors Are Coming to America for Health Care?" 2000. *Albany* (New York) *Times Union,* April 5, p. C8.

Iglehart, John. 1989. "The United States Looks at Canadian Health Care." *New England Journal of Medicine* 321(25): 1767–1772.

———. 2000a. "Revisiting the Canadian Health Care System." *New England Journal of Medicine* 342(26): 2007–2012.

———. 2000b. "Restoring the Status of an Icon: A Talk with Canada's Minister of Health." *Health Affairs* 19(3): 132–140.

Katz, Steven J., Diana Verrilli, and Morris L. Barer. 1998. "Canadians' Use of U.S. Medical Services." *Health Affairs* 17(1): 225–235.

Lassey, Marie L., William R. Lassey, and Martin J. Jinks. 1997. *Health Care Systems around the World: Characteristics, Issues, Reforms.* Upper Saddle River, NJ: Prentice-Hall.

Leatt, Peggy, and A. Paul Williams. 1997. "The Health System of Canada." In *Health Care and Reform in Industrialized Countries,* ed. Marshall W. Raffel. University Park: Pennsylvania State University Press.

Leslie, Donald R. 1997. "Health and Poverty in Canada." In *Health and Poverty,* ed. Michael J. Holosko and Marvin D. Feit. New York: Haworth Press.

Livingston, Martha. 1998. "Update on Health Care in Canada: What's Right, What's Wrong, What's Left." *Journal of Public Health Policy* 19(3): 267–288.

Lomas, Jonathan. 1997. "Devolving Authority for Health Care in Canada's Provinces: Emerging Issues and Prospects." *Canadian Medial Association Journal* 156(6): 817–823.

Lomas, Jonathan, John Woods, and Gerry Veenstra. 1997. "Devolving Authority for Health Care in Canada's Provinces: 1. An Introduction to the Issues." *Canadian Medical Association Journal* 156(3): 371–377.

Lomas, Jonathan, Gerry Veenstra, and John Woods. 1997. "Devolving Authority for Health Care in Canada's Provinces: 2. Backgrounds, Resources and Activities of Board Members." *Canadian Medical Association Journal* 156(4): 513–520.

Maioni, Antonia. 1998. *Parting at the Crossroads: The Emergence of Health Insurance in the United States and Canada*. Princeton, NJ: Princeton University Press.

Mhatre, Sharmila L., and Raisa B. Derber. 1998. "From Equal Access to Health Care to Equitable Access to Health: A Review of Canadian Provincial Health Commissions and Reports." In *Health and Canadian Society: Sociological Perspectives*, 3rd ed., ed. David Coburn, Carl D'Arcy, and George Torrance. Toronto: University of Toronto Press. (Originally published in *International Journal of Health Services*, 22(4): 645–668, 1992)

National Center for Health Statistics. 2000. *Health, United States, 2000*. Hyattsville, MD: Government Printing Office.

Naylor, C. David. 1999. "Health Care in Canada: Incrementalism under Fiscal Duress." *Health Affairs* 18(3): 9–26.

Organization for Economic Cooperation and Development. 1994. *The Reform of Health Care Systems: A Review of Seventeen OECD Countries*. Paris, France.
———. 2000. Health Data 2000. Paris, France.

Reamy, Jack. 1991. "Health Care in Canada: Lessons for the United States." *Journal of Rural Health* 7(3): 210–221.

Roemer, Milton I. 1991. *The Countries*. Vol. 1 of *National Health Care Systems of the World*. New York: Oxford University Press.

Roos, Noralou P., and Cameron A. Mustard. 1997. "Variation in Health and Health Care Use by Socioeconomic Status in Winnipeg, Canada: Does the System Work Well? Yes and No." *Milbank Quarterly* 75(1): 89–111.

Roos, Noralou P., Marni Brownell, Evelyn Shapiro, and Leslie L. Roos. 1998. "Good News about Difficult Decisions: The Canadian Approach to Hospital Cost Control." *Health Affairs* 17(5): 239–246.

Rozek, Richard, and Carla Mulhern. 1994. "The Health Care System in Canada." In *Financing Health Care*, Vol. 1, ed. Ullrich K. Hoffmeyer and Thomas R. McCarthy. Dordrecht: Kluwer Academic Publishers.

Sibbald, Barbara. 1998. "In Your Face: A New Wave of Militant Doctors Lashes Out." *Canadian Medical Association Journal* 158(11): 1505–1509.

Statistics Canada. 1999. *Statistical Report on the Health of Canadians*. Catalogue No. H39–467/199E. www.statcan.ca. August 20, 2000.

Swartz, Donald. 1998. "The Limits of Health Insurance." In *Health and Canadian Society: Sociological Perspectives*, 3rd ed., ed. David Coburn, Carl D'Arcy, and George Torrance. Toronto: University of Toronto Press.

Taylor, Malcolm G. 1986. "The Canadian Health Care System 1974–1984." In *Medicare at Maturity: Achievements and Challenges*, ed. Robert G. Evans and Greg L. Stoddart. Calgary, Alberta: University of Calgary Press.
———. 1990. *Insuring National Health Care: The Canadian Experience*. Chapel Hill: University of North Carolina Press.

Torrance, George M. 1998. "Socio-Historical Overview: The Development of the Canadian Health System." In *Health and Canadian Society: Sociological Perspectives*, 3rd ed., ed. David Coburn, Carl D'Arcy, and George Torrance. Toronto: University of Toronto Press.

U.S. Bureau of the Census. 1992. *International Population Reports*, P25, 92–3, An Aging World II. Washington, DC: Government Printing Office.

White, Joseph. 1995. *Competing Solutions: American Health Care Proposals and International Experience.* Washington, DC: The Brookings Institution.

Williams, A. Paul, Eugene Vayda, May L. Cohen, Christer A. Woodward, and Barbara M. Ferrier. 1995. "Medicine and the Canadian State: From the Politics of Conflict to the Politics of Accommodation." *Journal of Health and Social Behavior* 36(4): 303–321.

World Health Organization. 2000. *The World Health Report 2000. Health Systems: Improving Performance.* Geneva, Switzerland.

# CHAPTER 4

# United Kingdom

The principle that distinguishes a national health service from all other forms of medical and health care delivery is that it is a delivery system accountable, through the body politic, to the population it serves.

(Gill 1994: 455)

## INTRODUCTION

The preceding statement articulates the intent and focus of the British National Health Service (NHS). As we wend our way through the various health care systems in this book, we should note that the NHS has historically been characterized as "a health model for the entire world" (Roemer 1991: 191). Similarly, the NHS is "used by many countries as a 'model' of what a health system should desire to achieve" (Scheffler 1992: 180). At the same time, the NHS has been vilified for being underfinanced, overly centralized, and creating potentially life-threatening patient queues. Regardless of how the current system is assessed, the NHS, like all health care systems, emerged as the result of politically motivated interests as well as historically significant events (examined in the following section).

As with the Canadian system described in chapter 3, the NHS is located within the Beveridge model of health care systems. This model is characterized by "universal coverage for the country's residents, financing derived by national general taxes, and some form of national ownership/control of the factors of production" (Angus 1997: 26). In addition, the system provides free access at the point of delivery. According to Light

(1997), the NHS is perhaps best understood as the world's largest managed care organization.

The following pages outline the organizational structure and future of the NHS. I also address the differential impact of the NHS on the basis of age, sex, race and ethnicity, and social class. As always, the chapter begins with a historical overview.

## HISTORY OF THE NATIONAL HEALTH SERVICE

Although health care in England can be traced to the development of hospitals in the tenth century (Allen 1984), the National Health Service has its historical origins in the emergence of "friendly societies" during the nineteenth century. These societies are characterized as "a natural growth of associations of persons, often earning their livelihood in a similar fashion, who paid money into a common fund for some form of insurance purpose" (Lynch and Raphael 1963: 117). In addition to the friendly societies, the Poor Law Amendment Act of 1834 was intended to provide the poor and the sick with health care. As the industrial revolution progressed throughout the nineteenth century, rural populations were increasingly forced into urban centers. Because of this movement, the government became more concerned with public health issues such as sanitation. As a result, "a central authority—a central board of health under the Privy council" (U.S. Department of Health, Education and Welfare, 1976: 3) was established to address the increasing knowledge of disease patterns. The celebrated case of John Snow connecting the cause of death from cholera to the use of water from the Broad Street Pump illustrates such an effort.

Additional governmental efforts to legislate health directives occurred throughout the nineteenth and early twentieth centuries. Lloyd George, the Chancellor of the Exchequer, introduced the most important national legislation, the National Health Insurance Bill, in 1911. The legislation "mandated limited medical coverage for low-income workers" (Graig 1999: 154–155). The legislation angered workers because it required deductions from their pay (Cartwright 1977). The legislation, which persisted until the 1940s, was also criticized because it limited medical coverage to the worker and covered only services provided by general practitioners. Physicians, concerned that the available monies would not be fairly distributed, voted for a capitation method of payment for services (Roemer 1977).

The interwar years (1919–1939) experienced a variety of health initiatives that did not adequately address the problems inherent within the National Health Insurance Act. For example, insufficient funding, the lack of adequate facilities, and ongoing competition between voluntary and municipal hospitals are identified as systemic problems of the health care system prior to World War II. Furthermore, half of the population was not covered by health insurance in 1939 (Allen 1984). With the onset of World

War II, the British government created the Emergency Medical Service (EMS), whose purpose was to coordinate hospital beds throughout the country and cover the cost of casualties incurred as a result of the war. The inadequacy of hospitals, particularly those outside the major urban areas, became increasingly evident as the civilian population and medical staff was dispersed into the rural areas during the war (Allen 1984).

In the early 1940s, various political parties, as well as the British Medical Association, all developed permutations of a universal health care system. However, it was the work of Sir William Beveridge and others that culminated in the Beveridge Report in 1942, which outlined the framework of what would become the National Health Service. In addition to ensuring universal coverage, the newly created NHS provided "hospital treatment, freely available for the whole population and financed by insurance contributions" (Cartwright 1977: 173). Physicians, however, were less than enthusiastic about the NHS. As a result, concessions, such as allowing them to maintain private practice and not requiring them to become salaried civil servants, were included (Andrain 1998). Organizationally, the NHS consisted of "a tiered system of central administration, regional hospital boards, local health authorities and executive councils, and a tripartite of providers: hospital, community, and family practice services" (Lassey, Lassey, and Jinks 1997: 221). The bill creating the NHS was passed in 1946, but it was not officially implemented until July 5, 1948. The NHS is an entitlement that ensures a number of rights to UK citizens. These rights include the following:

- To be registered with a general practitioner (GP)
- To be referred to a consultant acceptable to him or her where the GP thinks it necessary; and
- To receive emergency medical care at any time. (Heppell 1994: 131)

Originally, the NHS was divided into three major components under the auspices of the minister of health: regional hospital boards, local health authorities, and executive councils (Figure 4.1). The 14 regional hospital boards (RHBs) in England were responsible for long-term policy, and the 330 hospital management committees (HMCs) in England and Wales were responsible for the daily management of the facilities. The 36 teaching hospitals were not under the control of RHBs, but rather boards of governors appointed by the secretary of state (Maynard 1975). Each hospital region contained between 2 and 3 million people and approximately 30,000 beds (Roemer, 1985). Second, local health professionals were paid by the 138 executive councils (ECs) in England and Wales to provide ambulatory services. For example, executive councils were responsible for capitation payments to GPs determined by the number of patients on their list, whereas dental services were paid on a fee-for-service basis. Initially, prescription drugs were completely covered. However, because of increasing drug

**Figure 4.1**
**The National Health Service in 1948**

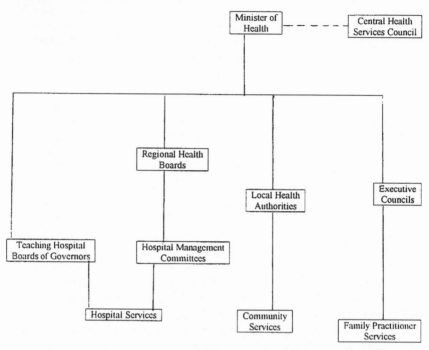

*Source:* Lassey, Marie L., William R. Lassey, and Martin J. Jinks. 1997. *Health Care Systems around the World: Characteristics, Issues, Reforms.* Figure 10.1. p. 222. Upper Saddle River, NJ: Prentice-Hall. HEALTH CARE SYSTEMS AROUND THE WORLD by Lassey & Lassey, © Reprinted with permission of Pearson Education, Inc., Upper Saddle River, NJ.

costs, a co-payment was initiated in the early 1950s (Roemer 1991). Finally, 146 local health authorities (LHAs) provided a variety of preventive and public health services ranging from postnatal care to home nursing. Local health authorities also created health centers that provided a range of services (see also O. Anderson 1972).

As with all health care systems, the NHS continues to experience structural change. The first major reorganization of the system occurred in 1974 with the objective of increasing the efficiency of service delivery. In the process, the three original components were to be "replaced by a structure of complete integration combining all these sectors into one comprehensive organization" (Ertler et al. 1987: 37). These reorganizational efforts resulted in the creation of regional health authorities (formerly the regional hospital boards) and area health authorities (formerly the local authorities). The executive councils remained but were put under the control of the Family

Practitioner Committee that was directly responsible to the Department of Health and Social Services (Barnard and Pendreigh 1982). The 90 area health authorities would be responsible for populations ranging from 250,000 to 1.5 million; the 14 regional health authorities would contain from 1 to 11 AHAs or some 1 to 5 million persons (Roemer 1985).

Further reorganization of the NHS occurred throughout the 1980s and 1990s. In 1982, the area health authorities (which were created in 1974) were eliminated (Organization for Economic Cooperation and Development 1992). Concomitantly, private health care opportunities increased through the efforts of the conservative Thatcher government. By the mid-1980s, 10% of the population was covered by private insurance.

According to Day and Klein (1989), the 1980s witnessed the emergence of four broad changes within the NHS. First, was a return to centralization, a style consistent with the Thatcher government. Increased centralization also represented an effort to make the NHS more accountable to Parliament for the money it spent. Centralization also shifted emphasis from inputs (number of beds, staff) to outputs (treatment of patients/operations, and so forth).

The second change was a new management style. A 1983 document by Roy Griffiths, director of a supermarket chain, outlined a management structure for the NHS. This structure would incorporate general managers at all levels of the NHS and reduce the role of doctors and nursing representatives in the decision-making process.

The third change involved an increased private sector within the health care community. Growth in this sector has been limited but consistent with social class position. Interestingly, the movement toward a larger role for the private sector has had the effect of solidifying the medical community's support for the NHS. Perhaps most important is the impact the private sector has had on long-term care. Here, the private, and voluntary, sector became the "largest producer of institutional long-stay care for the elderly by 1987" (Day and Klein 1989: 16).

The fourth change addressed efforts to control the gatekeepers (i.e., general practitioners). As Day and Klein (1989) point out, the NHS had never instituted control over general practitioners, even though they are the most responsible for deciding who receives care. Thus changes throughout the 1980s attempted to expand control over general practitioners via strengthened Family Practitioner Committees. It was anticipated that these committees would provide a managerial oversight of the quantity and quality of services provided by general practitioners. The goal of these committees was to "make general practitioners more sensitive to the preferences of their patients" (Day and Klein 1989: 20).

The most ambitious effort to reform the NHS since its inception is outlined in the 1989 white paper, *Working for Patients, 1989*. These reforms were the basis for the National Health Service and Community Care Act of

1990 that went into effect in 1991. Under the sponsorship of the Thatcher government, these reforms separated "the purchasing and provision of hospital services, mediated by contracts" (Organization for Economic Cooperation and Development 1992: 122). More specifically, the 1991 reforms can be categorized into three substantive areas: "separation of providers and purchasers; introduction of provider competition, and some choice of insurance coverage" (Hoffmeyer and Lloyd 1994: 99). The sources for financing the NHS were retained, however. Thus district health authorities, which previously provided those health services necessary for the population, now purchased, with a fixed budget, health services from those providers best able to meet their needs (Hart 1994; Ranade 1998).

At the same time, although hospitals remained public entities, they could become independent NHS Trusts competing for patients. They could also regulate their financial outcomes by determining employee pay scales, borrowing money, and creating surpluses. These hospitals were financed through contracts with health authorities and GP fundholders as well as through the sale of services to the private sector. The outcome was a system "based on competition between providers, with purchasers acting as proxy-consumers on behalf of their propulsions" (Klein 1995: 301). Competition between hospitals, however, is limited to their availability to a given population (Hatcher 1997).

Furthermore, the 1991 reforms altered the role of physicians by allowing individual general practitioners to form a larger GP practice that would become a fundholder. That is, the practice would not only receive their capitation fee for each patient on their list (between 1,000 and 1,500), but also an additional budget, allowing them to purchase services from providers (i.e., hospitals) on behalf of their patients (Holland and Graham 1994). Hospital services available for purchase by fundholders are "limited to elective surgical procedures and investigations generally costing less than 6,000 pounds" (Hatcher 1997: 235). Thus GP fundholders are, in reality, an HMO (Klein 1995).

The reforms associated with the 1991 legislation have had a significant impact on the NHS. But have the reforms resulted in increased efficiency of the system? According to many, the answer is no. Although the reforms have increased the percentage of health care costs associated with the bureaucracy of the system, there has not been a similar increase in the number of health professionals or their remuneration (Holland and Graham 1994). At the same time, the Organization for Economic Cooperation and Development (1992) suggests that GP fundholders appear to have improved their bargaining position (and power) relative to hospitals while strengthening the argument that they are skimming off the healthier patients in an effort to hold down costs. Others (for example, Ham 1996; Jacobs 1998; Mohan 1996) provide a range of interpretations regarding the

**Figure 4.2**
**Core Principles of the National Health Service**

- The NHS will provide a universal service for all based on clinical need, not ability to pay
- The NHS will provide a comprehensive range of services
- The NHS will shape its services around the needs and preferences of individual patients, their families and their careers
- The NHS will respond to different needs of different populations
- The NHS will work continuously to improve quality services and to minimise errors
- The NHS will support and value its staff
- Public funds for healthcare will be devoted solely to NHS patients
- The NHS will work together with others to ensure a seamless service for patients
- The NHS will help keep people healthy and work to reduce health inequalities
- The NHS will respect the confidentiality of individual patients and provide open access to information about services, treatment and performance

*Source:* The NHS Plan 2000: 3–5. Crown copyright material is reproduced with the permission of the Controller of HMSO and the Queen's Printer for Scotland.

reasons for and consequences of the 1991 *Working for Patients* reform efforts (see also Williams et al. 1993 for a review of NHS reforms during the 1980s).

The most current reforms are embedded in the recently released *NHS Plan* (2000). The following principles are from *The NHS Plan* (2000: 3–5) (see Figure 4.2). in which the secretary of state for health outlines "the common ground between the Government and the NHS" (*The NHS Plan* 2000: 3).

These principles provide a broad framework outlining the relationships among the government, patients, and health care providers. More importantly, these reform efforts will require continued infusion of additional financial support from the national government (see, for example, Morris 2000). Although the percentage of GDP spent on health care is expected to increase as a result of these reforms, critics have decried what they consider too little financial support, given the extensive needs of a health care system that for too long has been underfunded.

Finally, the year 2000 also witnessed the incorporation of the Human Rights Act 1998 in Great Britain. Some of the articles in this act are relevant to the health care of the population. For example, Article 2 states the right to life "shall be protected by law" (Horton 2000: 1186). Horton (2000) suggests that the wording in this article and others is vague, allowing for debate regarding intent. However, Horton criticizes the UK declaration as omitting articles found in the broader United Nations 1948 Universal Declaration. For example, Article 25 addresses the right to a standard of living that includes those necessities associated with maintaining health and well-being. Although these articles provide a framework within which rights are to be protected, they are also perceived as disconcerting because they give preference to individual rather than societal rights.

This brief historical excursion illustrates the strength and adaptability of the NHS. The following section examines more specifically the financing and delivery of health care services in the United Kingdom.

## FINANCING AND DELIVERY OF HEALTH CARE

As mentioned earlier, health care in the United Kingdom was originally financed through payroll deductions to cover the cost of basic services paid for by friendly societies. With the inception of the NHS in 1948, health care has been financed primarily from general taxes. Approximately 85% of health care expenditures are from public sources. The private sector provides services to 11% of the population and accounts for some 4% of expenditures (Smee 2000). Other sources, such as out-of-pocket expenses, constitute the remaining financing.

The United Kingdom spends roughly 6.7% of GDP, one of the lowest percentages in the industrialized world, to ensure health care for all its citizens. According to Rowlatt and Lloyd (1994), "the cabinet decides the sum that it wishes to spend on the NHS, and adjusts its policies to control total expenditure over time" (125). The ability of the UK to limit its level of health care spending and at the same time ensure universal coverage to all citizens represents governmental efforts to create a program that is, for the most part, financially prudent and socially responsible.

As alluded to earlier, the low levels of expenditures for the NHS have created some problems. The most pressing systemic problem has been the persistent underfunding of the NHS. Thus the crux of *The NHS Plan, 2000* is to infuse the NHS with much needed economic assistance. The level of health care spending is expected to increase by a third, from 50 to 69 billion pounds (Editorial 2000). The increased funding will improve the performance of the NHS, but questions persist regarding the government's commitment to these funding levels and differences over funding priorities. For example, an editorial ("The NHS Plan" 2000) in the *Lancet* argues that the plan fails to address adequately the needs of children and other vulnerable groups.

The lack of NHS funding has also created waiting lists for some services. As a result, some 10% of the population is covered by private insurance. Regarding utilization, research indicates that women are more likely than men to use the private health care sector because of the services offered (long-term stay, fertility clinics, and abortion services) (Wiles 1993). In addition, men and women reported different reasons for going private. For men, the main reason for going private was to reduce "disruption to their employment," whereas women identified the need to minimize "disruption at home" (Wiles 1993: 82–83). Although the percentage of the population covered by private health insurance increased throughout the 1980s and early 1990s, the current total has remained relatively constant. Furthermore, those covered with private insurance are not abandoning the NHS. Rather, they are utilizing the private sector in an effort to circumvent the need for queuing that is associated with various health-related services (Besley, Hall, and Preston 1998). However, a more insidious outcome of the private sector is the emergence of a two-tiered system. That is, those who can afford private health care would be less inclined to support a public (NHS) program (Jefferys 1992). Although it has been argued that competition between the public NHS and a private health care marketplace will improve efficiency of care, there is little empirical support. Rather, as Light (2000) suggests, "competition policy in health care, then, was and is used as a...set of rules and rewards that aim to get people and institutions to behave in cost-containing ways, and it shifts the responsibility for holding down costs to them" (971).

### Physicians

The primary route for the delivery of primary health care services is through an increasing number of general practitioners and other health care professionals controlled by the government through training and pay. During the nineteenth century, most general practitioners provided medical services while employed in solo practice or small groups (Larkin 1993). More recently, however, the number of GPs in partnerships of three or fewer has been decreasing, and the number in partnerships of six or more increased by 54% between 1988 and 1999. Doctors in fundholding practices provide services to over half the patient population (54%) (Department of Health 2000).

Medical practitioners in the NHS can be divided into two broad categories: general practitioners and consultant specialists. GPs provide office-based primary care services to the patients on their lists. General practitioners, who make house calls, are paid on a nationally established capitation formula with additional payments for treating specific services or populations (Hatcher 1997).

General practitioners are also more likely to be female, work part time, and have smaller lists. According to Department of Health (2000) statistics, 31% of doctors in 1998 were women, compared with 22% ten years earlier. Doctors who are female are also more likely to work part time or have more flexible work schedules. The average GP list has also decreased from 1,999 in 1988 to 1,866 in 1998. In addition to an overall increase in the number of doctors between 1988 and 1998 and an anticipated 20% increase in the medical school enrollment (Warden, 1998), there has also been a concomitant increase in the overall number of staff employed by doctors. The general increase in the number of doctors is being supplemented by some 2,000 refugee doctors who are being provided the necessary training to practice medicine in the NHS (Mayor 2000).

Specialists provide all hospital-based services. Previously, regional health authorities had paid specialists. With the 1991 reforms, specialists are now on contract (full or part time) with hospital trusts, although pay scales are standardized across the country for all fields (Hatcher 1997).

With a growing commitment to the profession of medicine, and increased organizational flexibility, the NHS is also establishing new rights and responsibilities for physicians (Richards 1998). There are concerns, however, that general practitioners have become less accessible to patients (Samuel 2000). Given the ongoing demographic shift toward an aging population, such concerns could become problematic for those citizens in need of continued contact with doctors.

### Hospitals

Construction of charity hospitals in the early 1700s provides a beginning point for the history of hospitals in England. When the NHS became operational in July 1948, the 2,700 hospitals in the UK became part of the system. At the time, many of the hospitals were experiencing financial difficulties that were ameliorated when the national government assumed control (Roemer 1991). Many of these hospitals, however, were physically dated. According to Allen (1984), "45 percent were erected before 1891 and 21 percent before 1861" (211). Because of limited finances, little hospital construction occurred in the early years of the NHS. In addition, hospitals and hospital beds were not distributed equally. Since the 1960s, however, efforts have been made to update hospitals throughout the system.

Hospitals under the NHS have undergone considerable reorganization since 1948 as a result of health reform efforts discussed earlier in the chapter. Nevertheless, one of the most contentious issues within the NHS has been the requisite queuing of patients as they wait their turn for many hospital-based services. Hospital waiting lists, however, existed prior to the development of the NHS. According to one study in the latter 1930s, some 100,000 patients had to wait for admission to voluntary hospitals (Lynch and Raphael 1963). Patient queuing has remained a significant problem, regardless of how health care is administered. More recently, efforts have attempted to increase the number of hospital beds and reduce the waiting time for admission (*The NHS Plan* 2000).

Comparing hospital statistics with other industrialized nations, Anderson (1998) reports that the UK was just above (16%) the OECD mean (15.9%) for hospital inpatient admission rates in 1996 and below (9.8) the OECD average of 10.6 for average length of hospital stay. At $320, the UK was well above the OECD average of $229 for per-day hospital costs.

Among the OECD countries included in his research, Anderson also reports that the UK was second only to the United States in terms of the number of acute care hospital staff per bed (3.5 and 3.8, respectively). In addition, Donelan et al. (1999) report that in comparison with respondents from Australia, Canada, New Zealand, and the United States, UK respondents were most likely to rate their overall hospital experience as excellent or good and considered their length of hospital stay as about right.

## CURRENT REALITIES AND THE ROLE OF THE STATE

Similar to the American and Canadian systems discussed earlier, the NHS continues to experience financial and organizational restructuring. For example, under the conservative governments of Margaret Thatcher and John Majors, efforts focused on creating an internal market in which the purchasing and provision of care would be separated, creating what Mechanic (1995) described as the Americanization of the NHS. Under the Labour government of Tony Blair, governmental spending on health care has increased substantially, but has also promulgated ongoing system reform (e.g., *The NHS Plan* 2000). These changes reflect not only the continuing influence of the political system on health policy but also demographic changes such as the aging of the population as well as increasing levels of technology. For example, the following statement in *The Lancet* "that patients and the NHS staff alike have been consistently ill-served by politicians of all parties" (Editorial 2000: 441) addresses not only the role of the state, but also its consequences relative to health opportunities and outcomes. Nevertheless, citizens in the UK are least likely to identify their health care system as in need of rebuilding (Donelan et al. 1999). And, as Light (1999) points out, "an equitable, universal health care system with a strong primary care base" (328) offers a number of valuable lessons for others.

Although the NHS is lauded for its successes and financial prudence, it has been consistently underfunded by the national government. Given the paucity of financial input into the system, the NHS is, nevertheless, ranked 18th in the world in terms of overall system performance (World Health Organization 2000). Also, because of limited resources, the NHS has utilized explicit rationing. That is, "some services are provided at the expense of others" (Kaufman 1994: 385). The infusion of additional spending by the Blair government has provided some financial relief to the system. However, the extra funding is intended to reduce the waiting time and the number of patients waiting for services as well as increase the number of hospital beds and physicians.

The UK and the other health care systems presented in this book share a number of common concerns for the future. They include controlling health care spending, managing the cost of hospital care, emphasizing primary care, containing the cost of medication, ensuring the quality of care, and reducing inequalities in access and services (President's Message 1998).

## THE HEALTH OF THE POPULATION BY AGE, SEX, SOCIAL CLASS, AND RACE AND ETHNICITY

The United Kingdom has experienced a significant increase in the life expectancy rates for males and females as well as a corresponding decline in the infant mortality rate. Currently, the life expectancy rate is 74.7 for males and 79.7 for females (World Health Organization 2000). The infant mortality rate declined from 22.5 in 1960 to 5.7 deaths per 1,000 live births in 1998 (Organization for Economic Cooperation and Development 2000).

Although the overall health of the population is improving, differences among segments of the population persist. According to Gabe (1997), access and use of health care remain unequal on the basis of class, gender, and race. Recently, official debate over this issue has depended on the government in power. Whitehead (1998) identifies significant dates in the historical progression of the debate. For example, in 1970, population health is identified as falling behind that of other European nations. Seven years later, the Labour government established the Inequalities in Health Research Working Group under Sir Douglas Black. In 1980, the working group published its findings, which stated that significant inequalities exist. The new conservative government of Margaret Thatcher, however, ignored the findings. In fact, by the mid-1980s, "any mention of health inequalities disappears from official vocabulary and statistics" (Whitehead 1998: 481). By the late 1990s, the newly elected Labour government identified efforts to reduce health inequalities as one of their major initiatives.

The inequalities in health in the UK on the basis of age, sex, social class, and race and ethnicity reflect the continued impact of inequalities in areas such as income, housing, job opportunities, and the environment (see, for example, Ramsay 1998). Furthermore, there is considerable overlap among these characteristics. Finally, the differential outcomes identified here should not be considered as evidence that the NHS has failed to achieve its objectives.

### Age

The population of the UK is becoming increasingly older. One hundred years ago, 4.7% of the population was age 65 or older. By 1981, the over-age-65 segment of the population had increased to 15% (Victor 1991). The over-age-65 population is projected to increase to 17.1% in 2010 and 21.5% in 2025 (U.S. Bureau of the Census 1992). According to Anderson and Hussey (1999), a 65-year-old female could expect to live an additional 18.3

years and a male 14.8 years. Typical of other industrialized nations, the majority of the over-65 population is female. Although the percentage of the over-65 population residing in an institutional setting is relatively low, the residents are far more likely to be female than male. In addition, the percentage of older adults reporting good health status decreased from 79.5% in 1998 to 77.1% in 1998. During the same time period, the percentage of older females and males reporting good health status decreased from 77.9% to 75.5% and 82.0% to 79.2%, respectively (Organization for Economic Cooperation and Development 2000).

Efforts have been made to improve the quality of life for an increasingly aging population, but discrimination on the basis of age continues. Age discrimination has been of particular concern ever since Aaron and Schwartz (1984) and Halper (1989) argued that older citizens are less likely than younger citizens to receive dialysis treatment. And, "unless age-rationing is explicitly prohibited, the BNHS will continue to distribute resources inequitably" (Baker 1993: 149). Evans (1997) points out that older citizens also receive less than adequate treatment for problems of the heart such as acute myocardial infarction. In addition, differential outcomes within existing programs generally benefit males over females, those who are economically advantaged rather than the poor, and whites over minority elderly (Lassey and Lassey 2001). In comparison with other industrialized nations (Australia, Canada, New Zealand, and the United States), the elderly in the UK report that access to needed medical care, specialists, and nonemergency surgery is more difficult. However, in comparison with elderly in the same industrialized nations, the elderly in the UK report the lowest level of out-of-pocket expenses for prescription drugs, the highest perceived health status, and the least difficulty paying medical bills (Schoen et al. 2000).

Attempting to address one of the most expensive problems of growing older, the national government will begin treating long-term care "the same as care elsewhere in the NHS—free at the point of use" (Beecham 2000: 318). Between 1980 and 1990, use of primarily private sector long-term care (nursing homes) increased 41%, and residential care home use increased 48% (Lassey and Lassey 2001). At the same time, there have been ongoing efforts to expand alternatives to institutionalization, such as community care (Department of Health 1999a). Unfortunately, the demand for community care has generally been significantly greater than the resources available (Cox 1997). Regardless of the type of care provided, paid care for the aging population increased 34% between 1992 and 1998 (Ungerson 2000). The characteristics of institutionalized patients depend on the type of long-term care facility. For instance, nursing home residents are typically widowed or single females in their early 80s, whereas residents in hospital long-term-stay facilities are more likely to be married men (Victor 1991).

It appears that an aging population and the governmental desire to control health care costs could prove a difficult balancing act. On the one hand, the government is increasing its financial commitment to meet the general social and health service needs of an aging population; on the other, there remains the potential for continued rationing of potentially livesaving care on the basis of age. This is of particular concern for low-income and minority elderly.

### Sex

Differential health outcomes on the basis of sex are not unique to the United Kingdom. The research indicates that as in other industrialized nations, women outlive men in the United Kingdom (Sidell 1995). Women are also more likely than men to experience chronic health problems (Victor 1991). Similarly, older women are more likely than older men to experience disability and limited mobility. Men, however, are more likely to die at an earlier age (Lassey and Lassey 2001). Furthermore, Jordan, Ong, and Croft (2000) report that limiting long-term illnesses are related not only to age but also sex. According to Jordan et al. (2000), males are most likely to experience limiting long-term illnesses between the ages of 50 and 64, and women experience such problems after the age of 65.

Examining why one-third of males over the age of 50 in the United Kingdom have prostate conditions, Cameron and Bernardes (1998) identify a number of assumptions about men's health that include "health is women's, not men's business and responsibility; men know little about men's health; men tend to keep quiet about their health problems; health/health promotion is 'female' so being a man means being denied a self-monitoring role; and prostate problems represent a threat to masculinity/the self" (120–122). Given these assumptions, gender-based health outcomes are not surprising. However, Shaw, Dorling and Brimblecombe (1998) report that, regardless of area of country, excess mortality rates between males and females are relatively similar.

### Social Class

Health inequalities on the basis of social class have been collected for 150 years in Great Britain (Whitehead 1998). Utilizing the most recent findings from the Health Inequalities Decennial Supplement, Scott-Samuel (1997) argues that life expectancy differences of male and female infants born to semiskilled and unskilled laborers compared with professionals are 3 and 5 years less, respectively. Similarly, Mayor (1998) reports that the mortality rate among unskilled males was almost three times greater than the mortality rate for professional males, and Lahelma et al. (2000) suggest that inequalities in health are related to employment status.

Approaching this argument from a slightly different perspective, Wilkinson (1990) argues that life expectancy in developed nations increases as income distribution decreases. Thus there is little disagreement regarding the existence of the relationship between social class and health outcomes (see also Gray 1999). Rather, arguments have focused on attempting to explain why it exists. As a result, this section examines the publication and response to *The Black Report* (Townsend and Davidson 1992).

In 1977, the secretary of state for health created a working group on health inequalities. Consisting of four members, their task was to examine information regarding health differences among social classes, as well as their causes and implications. When completed, the incoming conservative Thatcher government attempted to suppress the release of the report.

Essentially, the report argued that after three decades of universal health care, differences in health outcomes among social classes remained. In addition, "organized health services can benefit health, but favorable living and working conditions can benefit health even more" (Roemer 1991: 205). In response to the causes of the continued health inequities, the report identified four possible explanations: artifact, natural/social selection, materialist/structural, and cultural/behavioral.

The artifact explanation suggests that social class and mortality are not related. Rather, Townsend and Davidson (1992: 105) suggest that health inequalities exist because of "the reduction in the proportion of the population in the poorest occupational classes." Furthermore, the "explanation recognises that the way social class or health is measured might influence the apparent magnitude of, and trends in, observed inequalities in health" (Macintyre 1997: 727).

The natural/social selection explanation argues there is a relationship between social class and health. Within this relationship it is understood that a person's social class is determined by his or her health. This explanation utilizes the drift hypothesis. In other words, those in the lower or upper social classes are there because of their health (they have drifted down or up the socioeconomic ladder). Vagero and Illsley (1995) suggest that the authors of *The Black Report* were unclear in their intentions regarding this explanation when they introduced it "and then dismiss genetic explanations for health inequalities, and in so doing also dismiss the social selection explanations" (223).

Materialist/structural explanation suggests that health differentials are the result of a person's class standing determined by his or her occupational status. In addition, this explanation argues that the relative deprivation creating class differentials is also responsible for health differentials. Thus the fundamental explanation for health inequality lies in the distribution of wealth and income within society.

Cultural/behavioral explanation is similar to the materialist/structural explanation. However, this argument locates the primary responsibility for the differential between social position and health within individual behavior rather the larger society (a culture of poverty approach). For instance, behaviors such as "smoking, poor diet, inappropriate use of health services" (Macintyre 1997: 728) and so forth, are identified as the primary explanation.

Given the four explanations, the authors of *The Black Report* considered the materialist or structuralist argument the strongest. Furthermore, the authors identified a number of priorities within health care, social policy, and research. Health care priorities consisted of the following:

- For children to have a better start in life;
- For disabled people bearing the brunt of cumulative ill health and deprivation; and
- For preventive and educational action to encourage good health;

Social policy includes the following:

- A comprehensive antipoverty strategy; and
- Improving education;

Research priorities consist of the following:

- Surveillance of the development of children, especially in relation to accidents;
- Better understanding of the health effects of such aspects of behavior as smoking, diet, alcohol consumption, and exercise;
- The development of area social conditions and health indicators for use in resource allocation;
- Study of health hazards in relation to occupational conditions and work;
- Better measures of the prevalence and course of disability; and
- Study of the interaction of social factors implicated in ill health over time and within small areas. (Macintyre 1997: 729–730)

Beginning in the mid-1980s, the work of David Barker and others attempted to further the relation between health and social class. The basis of their argument was that past poverty led to "programming during foetal and infant life as the most important determinant of social differences in adult health" (Vagero and Illsley 1995: 220). Although the work of Barker and others has been criticized, Vagero and Illsley (1995) identify some positive aspects of their work. For example, rather than examining biological programming as Barker did, they suggest an analysis of social programming that "is intended to sum up those social influences in early life which directly or indirectly determine adult health or which interact with adult experience to determine adult health" (Vagero and Illsley 1995: 231).These efforts are instructive because they attempt to broaden the understanding of the relationship between social class and health. Of particular importance in this discussion is the inclusion of the life course (see also van de Mheen et al. 1998).

### Race and Ethnicity

The population of the United Kingdom is primarily white. In the early 1990s, ethnic minorities constituted approximately 6% of the total population. Similar to other industrialized nations, differential health outcomes exist on the basis of race and ethnicity as well as social class. For example, Davey Smith (2000), in an analysis of the complex relationship between socioeconomic class and ethnicity, reports that mortality differences exist between manual and nonmanual laborers born in various countries of Africa, the Caribbean, and the Far East. According to the Department of Health (1999b), infant mortality rates among children of mothers from Pakistan and the Caribbean Commonwealth are double the national average. Atri et al. (1996) report similar findings. They found that ethnic minorities, particularly those from Bangladesh, are less likely to be employed or own a home or car. Furthermore, Curtis and Lawson (2000) state that the health behaviors and beliefs of minority populations may also differ. As a result, differential health outcomes on the basis of ethnicity are attributable not only to social class, but also culture. Jovchelovitch and Gervais (1999) point out "the cultural traditions of the Chinese community are key factors in the process of production, maintenance and reproduction of representations of health and illness" (259). The Health Survey for England (1999) also reports that self-assessed health among minorities, particularly Pakistani and Bangladeshi men and women, are far more likely to identify their health as bad or very bad compared with the general population.

Although access to health care is universal in the United Kingdom, minority populations experience greater difficulty receiving health-related services. As Bayne-Smith (1999) reports, "minorities must also deal with the additional obstacles of racism, discrimination, language and communication barriers which are also entrenched characteristics of the health care system as an institution" (179). Research by Staniszewska, Ahmed, and Jenkinson (1999), however, reveals little difference between white and Indian cardiac respondents regarding health differences. The authors qualify their findings by noting that the Indian respondents had lived in the UK for at least ten years and were considered well acculturated.

Research on age, sex, social class, and race and ethnicity relative to health in the United Kingdom reveals a complex interrelationship. Although research addresses the growing health inequalities within the UK, it is important to understand these outcomes as the result of a multiplicity of respondent characteristics. Thus efforts to reduce these differences must focus on issues such as living environments, occupations, and income as well as access to health care.

## CONCLUSION

Health care in the United Kingdom has undergone continued refinement since the development of friendly societies in the nineteenth century. During this period of time, various historical events have influenced the shift of health care responsibility from the individual to the state. In particular, the advent of World War II provided the impetus for an examination of British health care. In the early 1940s, Sir William Beveridge outlined what would eventually become the National Health Service in July 1948. The purpose of the NHS was to provide universal health care to all citizens in the UK. The NHS also ensured access to a general practitioner, referral to specialists when necessary, and the right to emergency treatment. Initially the NHS was divided into three components: regional hospital boards, local health authorities, and executive councils.

Since 1948, the NHS has been the object of numerous reform efforts. Beginning in 1974, the organizational structure was redesigned to include regional health authorities rather than the regional hospital boards, and area health authorities replaced local health authorities. By 1982, the area health authorities were eliminated. The early 1980s also witnessed governmental efforts to increase the private health care sector. Perhaps the most significant reform effort occurred with the *Working for Patients, 1989* white paper that eventually became the National Health Service and Community Care Act of 1991. Basically, this act separated purchasers and providers and created competition among providers with the creation of hospital trusts and physician fundholders. The impact of these reforms is still being evaluated. Meanwhile, the most recent reform efforts come out of the recently released *NHS Plan* (2000). In particular, these reforms are intended to raise the level of governmental spending on the NHS, thus providing for an increase in the number of physicians as well as hospital beds.

Although the NHS ensures universal access to care, particularly at the primary health level, inequalities persist. Examining the population by age, sex, social class, and race and ethnicity reveals particularly disturbing trends. In particular, these trends indicate that for some procedures, health care access is limited on the basis of age. Differential health outcomes also exist between males and females as well as the majority ethnic and an increasing ethnic minority population. Perhaps the most highly publicized health care outcomes are on the basis of social class position. Here, the publication of *The Black Report* in 1980 revealed increased health inequities between those populations in the lower and upper echelons of UK society (as measured by occupation). *The Black Report* argued that in addition to health care, other factors including the physical and social environment led to the increase in health outcomes. Although the conservative Thatcher government attempted to suppress the report, it was nevertheless made public.

Given the historical development and subsequent reforms, the NHS is a reminder that government can create and efficiently operate its health care system. Although per capita spending on the NHS is half what the United States spends, gross indicators of health indicate that members of the UK are as healthy as Americans. Furthermore, the World Health Organization has ranked the overall performance of the NHS as 18th in the world. By comparison, the United States health care system is ranked 35th overall. For all of its flaws, the NHS is not only a bargain, but also an inspiration.

## REFERENCES

Aaron, Henry, and William B. Schwartz. 1984. *The Painful Prescription.* Washington, DC: Brookings Institution.

Allen, David. 1984. "Health Services in England." In *Comparative Health Systems: Descriptive Analyses of Fourteen National Health Systems,* ed. Marshall W. Raffel. University Park: Pennsylvania State University Press.

Anderson, Gerard F. 1998. *Multinational Comparisons of Health Care: Expenditures, Coverage, and Outcomes.* New York: The Commonwealth Fund.

Anderson, Gerard F., and Peter S. Hussey. 1999. "Health and Population Aging: A Multinational Comparison." New York: The Commonwealth Fund.

Anderson, Odin W. 1972. *HEALTH CARE: Can There Be Equity? The United States, Sweden and England.* New York: John Wiley.

Andrain, Charles F. 1998. *Public Health Policies and Social Inequality.* New York: New York University Press.

Angus, Douglas E. 1997. "Health Care Costs: Canada in Perspective." In *Health and Canadian Society: Sociological Perspectives,* 3rd ed., ed. David Coburn, Carl D'Arcy, and George Torrance. Toronto: University of Toronto Press.

Atri, J., M. Falshaw, A. Livingstone, and J. Robson. 1996. "Fair Shares in Health Care? Ethnic and Socioeconomic Influences on Recording of Preventive Care in Selected Inner London General Practices." *British Medical Journal* 312: 614–619.

Baker, Robert. 1993. "Visibility and the Just Allocation of Health Care: A Study of Age-Rationing in the British National Health Service." *Health Care Analysis* 1(2): 139–150.

Barnard, Keith, and David Pendreigh. 1982. "The Health Services System of the United Kingdom." In *Reorienting Health Services: Application of a Systems Approach,* ed. Charles O. Pannenborg, Albert van der Werff, Gary B. Hirsch, and Keith Barnard. NATO Advanced Research Institute on Health Services Systems. Hague, Netherlands: Plenum Press.

Bayne-Smith, Marcia. 1999. "Primary Care: Choices and Opportunities for Racial/Ethnic Minority Populations in the USA and UK—A comparative analysis." *Ethnicity & Health* 4(3): 165–188.

Beecham, Linda. 2000. "Elderly People Will Get Free Nursing Care." *British Medical Journal* 321: 318.

Besley, Timothy, John Hall, and Ian Preston. 1998. "Private and Public Health Insurance in the UK." *European Economic Review* 42: 491–497.

Cameron, Elaine, and Jon Bernardes. 1998. "Gender and Disadvantage in Health: Men's Health for a Change." In *The Sociology of Health Inequalities,* ed. Mel Bartley, David Blane, and George Davey Smith. Oxford, UK: Blackwell.

Cartwright, F. F. 1977. *A Social History of Medicine.* London: Longman.

Cox, Carole. 1997. "Long-Term Care: A Comparison of Policies and Services in Israel and the United Kingdom and Implications for the United States." *Journal of Aging & Social Policy* 9(2): 81–99.

Curtis, Sarah, and Kim Lawson. 2000. "Gender, Ethnicity and Self-Reported Health: The Case of African-Caribbean Populations in London." *Social Science & Medicine* 50(3): 365–385.

Davey-Smith, George. 2000. "Learning to Live with Complexity: Ethnicity, Socio-economic Position, and Health in Britain and the United States." *American Journal of Public Health* 90(11): 1694–1698.

Day, Patricia, and Rudolf Klein. 1989. "The Politics of Modernization: Britain's National Health Service in the 1980's." *Milbank Quarterly* 67(1): 1–34.

Department of Health. 1999a. *Long Term Care: The Government's Response to the Health Committee's Report on Long Term Care.* London: Her Majesty's Stationary Office.

———. 1999b. *Reducing Health Inequalities: An Action Report.* London: Her Majesty's Stationary Office.

———. 2000. Statistics for General Medical Practitioners in England: 1988–1998. www.doh.gov.uk/public/medprac88–98.html. (May 8, 2000).

Donelan, Karen, et al. 1999. "The Cost of Health System Change: Public Discontent in Five Nations." *Health Affairs* 18(3): 206–216.

Ertler, Wolfgang, H. Schmidt, J. M. Treyth, and H. Wintersberger. 1987. "The Social Dimensions of Health and Health Care: An International Comparison." *Research in the Sociology of Health Care* 5: 1–62.

Evans, J. Grimley. 1997. "The Rationing Debate: Rationing Health Care by Age: The Case Against." *British Medical Journal* 314: 822–825.

Gabe, Johnathan. 1997. "Continuity and Change in the British National Service." In *The Sociology of Health & Illness: Critical Perspectives,* 5th ed., ed. Peter Conrad. New York: St. Martin's.

Gill, Derek. 1994. "A National Health Service: Principles and Practice." In *The Sociology of Health and Illness: Critical Perspectives,* 4th ed., ed. Peter Conrad and Rochelle Kern. New York: St. Martin's.

Graig, Laurene A. 1999. *Health of Nations: An International Perspective on U.S. Health Care Reform,* 3rd ed. Washington, DC: Congressional Quarterly.

Gray, Alastair. 1999. "Explaining Inequalities in Health in the United Kingdom." In *World Health and Disease,* ed. Alastair Gray. Buckingham, UK: Open University Press.

Halper, T. 1989. *The Misfortunes of Others: End-Stage Renal Disease in the United Kingdom.* Cambridge: Cambridge University Press.

Ham, Chris. 1996. "Population-Centered and Patient-Focused Purchasing: The U.K. Experience." *Milbank Quarterly* 74(2): 191–214.

Hart, Graham. 1994. "The NHS: Founding Principles and the Reforms." In *Health Care Systems in Canada & the United Kingdom*, ed. Kenneth Lee. Keele, UK: Ryburn Publishing.

Hatcher, Peter R. 1997. "The Health System of the United Kingdom." In *Health Care and Reform in Industrialized Countries*, ed. Marshall W. Raffel. University Park: Pennsylvania State University Press.

Health Survey for England. (1999). The Health of Minority Ethnic Groups. http://www.official-documents.co.uk/documents/doh/survey99/hses01.html. (May 15, 2001).

Heppell, Strachan. 1994. "The Future and Long-Range Planning of Health Care Services: UK." In *Health Care Systems in Canada & the United Kingdom: Can They Deliver?* ed. Kenneth Lee. Keele, UK: Ryburn Publishing.

Hoffmeyer, Ulrich, and Adam Lloyd. 1994. "Health Care Systems in Canada and the United Kingdom: Common Problems, Common Solutions?" In *Health Care Systems in Canada & the United Kingdom: Can They Deliver?* ed. Kenneth Lee. Keele, UK: Ryburn Publishing.

Holland, Walther W., and Clifford Graham. 1994. "Commentary: Recent Reforms in the British National Health Service—Lessons for the United States." *American Journal of Public Health* 84(2): 186–189.

Horton, Richard. 2000. "Health and the UK Human Rights Act 1998." *The Lancet* 356: 1186–1188.

Jacobs, Alan. 1998. "Seeing Difference: Market Health Reform in Europe." *Journal of Health Politics, Policy and Law* 23(1): 1–33.

Jefferys, Margot. 1992. "Britain's National Health Service under Pressure." In *Health Care Systems And Their Patients: An International Perspective*, ed. Marilynn M. Rosenthal and Marcel Frenkel. Boulder, CO: Westview Press.

Jordan, Kelvin, Bie Nio Ong, and Peter Croft. 2000. "Researching Limiting Long-Term Illness." *Social Science and Medicine* 50(3): 397–405.

Jovchelovitch, Sandra, and Marie-Claude Gervais. 1999. "Social Representations of Health and Illness: The Case of the Chinese Community in England." *Journal of Community & Applied Social Psychology* 9: 247–260.

Kaufman, Caroline. 1994. "Rights and the Provision of Health Care: A Comparison of Canada, Great Britain, and the United States." In *Dominant Issues in Health Care*, 3rd ed., ed. Howard D. Schwartz. New York: McGraw-Hill.

Klein, Rudolf. 1995. "Big Bang Health Care Reform—Does It Work?: The Case of Britain's 1991 National Health Service Reforms." *Milbank Quarterly* 73(3): 299–337.

Lahelma, Eero, Sara Arber, Ossi Rahkonen, and Karri Silventoinea. 2000. "Widening or Narrowing Inequalities in Health? Comparing Britain and Finland from the 1980s to the 1990s." *Sociology of Health & Illness* 22(1): 110–136.

Larkin, Gerald V. 1993. "Continuity in Change: Medical Dominance in the United Kingdom." In *The Changing Medical Profession: An International Perspective*, ed. Frederic W. Hafferty and John B. McKinlay. New York: Oxford.

Lassey, Marie L., William R. Lassey, and Martin J. Jinks. 1997. *Health Care Systems around the World: Characteristics, Issues, Reforms*. Upper Saddle River, NJ: Prentice-Hall.

Lassey, William R., and Marie L. Lassey. 2001. *Quality of Life for Older People: An International Perspective*. Upper Saddle River, NJ: Prentice-Hall.

Light, Donald W. 1997. "From Managed Competition to Managed Cooperation: Theory and Lessons from the British Experience." *Milbank Quarterly* 75(3): 297–340.

———. 1999. "Policy Lessons from the British Health Care System." In *Health Care Systems in Transition: An International Perspective,* ed. Francis D. Powell and Albert F. Wessen. Thousand Oaks, CA: Sage.

———. 2000. "Sociological Perspectives on Competition in Health Care." *Journal of Health Politics, Policy and Law* 25(5): 969–974.

Lynch, Matthew J., and Stanley S. Raphael. 1963. *Medicine and the State.* Springfield, IL: Charles C. Thomas.

Macintyre, Sally. 1997. "The Black Report and Beyond. What Are the Issues?" *Social Science and Medicine* 44(6): 723–745.

Maynard, Alan. 1975. *Health Care in the European Community.* Pittsburgh: University of Pittsburgh Press.

Mayor, Susan. 1998. "UK Report Calls for Policies to Halt Growing Inequalities in Health." *The Lancet* 317: 1471.

———. 2000. "UK Helps Refugee Doctors to Practice in NHS." *British Medical Journal* 321: 1178.

Mechanic, David. 1995. "The Americanization of the British National Health Service." *Health Affairs* 14(2): 51–67.

Mohan, John. 1996. "Accounts of the NHS Reforms: Macro-, Meso- and Micro Level Perspectives." *Sociology of Health and Illness* 18(5): 675–698.

Morris, Kelly. 2000. "Patient-Power Rules in New NHS." *The Lancet* 356: 487.

Organization for Economic Cooperation and Development. 1992. *The Reform of Health Care: A Comparative Analysis of Seven OECD Countries.* Paris, France.

———. 2000. OECD Health Data 2000. Paris, France.

President's Message. 1998. "Common Concerns: International Issues in Health Care System Reform." New York: Commonwealth Fund.

Ramsay, Sarah. 1998. "Remedy Presented for Health Inequalities in England." *The Lancet* 352: 1759.

Ranade, Wendy. 1998. "Reforming the British National Health Service: All Change, No Change?" In *Markets and Health Care: A Comparative Analysis,* ed. Wendy Ranade. London: Longman.

Richards, Peter. 1998. "Professional Self-Respect: Rights and Responsibilities in the New NHS." *British Medical Journal* 317: 1146–1148.

Roemer, Milton I. 1977. *Comparative National Policies on Health Care.* New York: Marcel Dekker.

———. 1985. *National Strategies for Health Care Organization: A World Overview.* Ann Arbor, MI: Health Administration Press.

———. 1991. *The Countries.* Vol. 1 of *National Health Systems of the World.* New York: Oxford.

Rowlatt, Penelope, and Adam Lloyd. 1994. "Projections of Health Care Need and Funding." In *Financing Health Care,* Vol. 1, ed. Ullrich K. Hoffmeyer and Thomas R. McCarthy. Dordrecht: Kluwer Academic Publishers.

Samuel, Oliver. 2000. "Is General Practice Losing Its Way?" *British Journal of Medicine* 321: 1421.

Scheffler, Richard M. 1992. "Culture versus Competition: The Reforms of the British National Health Service." *Journal of Public Health Policy* 13(2): 180–185.

Schoen, Cathy, Erin Strumpf, Karen Davis, Robin Osborn, Karen Donelan, and
    Robert J. Blendon. 2000. "The Elderly's Experiences with Health Care in
    Five Nations: Findings from the Commonwealth Fund 1999 International
    Health Policy Survey." New York: Commonwealth Fund.
Scott-Samuel, Alex. 1997. "Health Inequalities Recognized in UK." *The Lancet* 350:
    753.
Shaw, Mary, Danny Dorling, and Nic Brimblecombe. 1998. "Changing the Map:
    Health in Britain 1951–1991." In *The Sociology of Health Inequalities,* ed.
    Mel Bartley, David Blane, and George Davey Smith. Oxford, UK: Black-
    well.
Sidell, Moyra. 1995. *Health in Old Age: Myth, Mystery and Management.* Bucking-
    ham, UK: Open University Press.
Smee, Clive. 2000. "United Kingdom." *Journal of Health Politics, Policy and Law*
    25(5): 945–952.
Staniszewska, S., L. Ahmed, and C. Jenkinson. 1999. "The Conceptual Validity and
    Appropriateness of Using Health-Related Quality of Life Measures with
    Minority Ethnic Groups." *Ethnicity & Health* 4(1): 51–63.
*The NHS Plan: A Plan for Investment, A Plan for Reform.* 2000. Presented to Parlia-
    ment by the Secretary of State for Health by Command of Her Majesty. July
    2000. Printed in the UK for The Stationary Office Limited on Behalf of the
    Controller of Her Majesty's Stationary Office. Norwich, UK: Copyright, Her
    Majesty's Stationary Office.
"The NHS Plan: Promises That Fail the Most Vulnerable." 2000. Editorial. *The
    Lancet* 356: 441.
Townsend, P., and Davidson, N. 1992. *"Inequalities in Health: The Black Report."* Lon-
    don: Penguin.
Ungerson, Clare. 2000. "Thinking about the Production and Consumption of
    Long-Term Care in Britain: Does Gender Still Matter?" *Journal of Social Pol-
    icy* 29(4): 623–643.
U.S. Bureau of the Census. 1992. International Population Reports. P25, 92–3, *An
    Aging World II.* Washington, DC: Government Printing Office.
U.S. Department of Health, Education and Welfare. 1976. *The British National
    Health Service: Conversations with Sir George E. Godber.* Washington, DC: Gov-
    ernment Printing Office.
Vagero, Denny, and Raymond Illsley. 1995. "Explaining Health Inequalities:
    Beyond Black and Barker." *European Sociological Review* 11(3): 219–241.
van de Mheen, H. Dike, Karien Stronks, and Johann P. Mackenbach. 1998. "A Life-
    course Perspective on Socio-Economic Inequalities in Health: The Influence
    of Childhood Socio-Economic Conditions and Selection Processes." In *The
    Sociology of Health Inequalities,* ed. Mel Bartley, David Blane, and George
    Davey Smith. Oxford, UK: Blackwell.
Victor, Christina R. 1991. *Health and Health Care in Later Life.* Buckingham, UK:
    Open University Press.
Warden, John. 1998. "Extra 1000 Medical School Places by 2005." *The Lancet* 317:
    300.
Whitehead, Margaret. 1998. "Diffusion of Ideas on Social Inequalities in Health: A
    European Perspective." *Milbank Quarterly* 76(3): 469–492.
Wiles, Rose. 1993. "Women and Private Medicine." *Sociology of Health & Illness*
    15(1): 68–85.

Wilkinson, Richard G. 1990. "Income Distribution and Mortality: A 'Natural' Experiment." *Sociology of Health and Illness* 12(4): 391–412.

Williams, S. J., M. Calnan, S. L. Cant, and J. Coyle. 1993. "All Change in the NHS? Implications of the NHS Reforms for Primary Care Prevention." *Sociology of Health & Illness* 15(1): 43–67.

World Health Organization. 2000. *Health Systems: Improving Performance.* Geneva, Switzerland.

# CHAPTER 5

# Germany

The German government ensures that all working persons and their dependents have the most comprehensive, high quality health insurance benefits.
The plans provide for all inpatient and ambulatory care diagnostic and therapeutic services that are considered necessary and medically feasible. Tertiary services, such as heart transplants, are covered with a minimum
coinsurance payment. Some plans even provide two weeks at a spa every
other year for rehabilitation, if recommended by a physician.

(Weil 1992: 535)

## INTRODUCTION

This chapter locates the origins of the relationship between national government and health care in the German system. As the preceding quote
articulates, the German health care system represents the initial foray of
national government into the health care issue.

Distinct from the Beveridge model of health care represented by the systems in Canada and the United Kingdom, German health care is best
understood as social insurance, or the Bismarck model. Angus (1998) characterizes this system as "compulsory universal coverage within a social
security framework, [financed] by employer and individual contributions
through non-profit insurance funds, and a combination of public/private
ownership of the factors of production" (26). Organizationally, the German
health care system represents a middle ground between the entrepreneurial
American health care system and the government-controlled National

Health Service in the United Kingdom. The German system "combines the use of market-style incentives with indirect (regulations) and direct (financial) government involvement" (Pfaff and Wassener 2000: 910). The German system is also referred to as a corporatist model. In other words, the role of the government is that of referee among the various players in the health care system. As Light (1997) points out, the goal is to join "together employers, employees, physicians, hospitals, and other providers so that they must negotiate a budget for the medical costs of next year's illnesses" (477).

Originating in Germany in the mid-1880s, the national social insurance program offers a unique blend of private and public involvement in health care. The result has been a health care system that is considered one of the most comprehensive in the world. Most recently, the World Health Organization (2000) ranked the German system 25th internationally in overall system performance. Furthermore, until reunification, the German health care system had been able to contain increases in health care costs within the yearly growth rate of its gross domestic product (Iglehart 1991a). With unification, the German health care system experienced significant cost increases as former East Germans were integrated into the system. As a result, Germany has again instituted reform efforts to control health care spending. Nevertheless, the German health care system enjoys broad public support. For example, Blendon et al. (1990, 1995) found that only 13% of West Germans agreed that the health care system needed to be completely rebuilt, and 41% indicated only minor changes were necessary. Five years later, 11% stated that the system needed to be completely rebuilt; 30% agreed that the health care system only needed minor repairs. The most significant change occurred among those who believed the health care system is good, but in need of fundamental changes. In 1990, 35% of the respondents agreed; 55% agreed in 1995. Although such data indicate a weakening of public confidence in the system, Germans are far more supportive of their health care system than are Americans.

## HISTORY OF THE GERMAN HEALTH CARE SYSTEM

The German health care system emerged out of the political fervor of the mid- to late 1800s. With industrialization forcing the movement of rural populations to urban centers, worker discontent was growing, as was socialism. Concerned with the rise of political dissidence among workers, the politically conservative German chancellor, Otto von Bismarck, convinced Parliament in 1878 to control the political influence of socialist parties. Believing such action was not sufficient to quell worker unrest, Bismarck introduced the Sickness Insurance Act in 1881 (Roemer 1991). The purpose of the bill was to provide a national sickness fund for low-wage workers. The act was passed in 1883 and took effect on December 1, 1884 (Lynch and Raphael 1963).

By 1885, there were some 5,000 sickness funds covering over 4 million workers, approximately one-sixth of whom were women. The number of sickness funds continued to expand until the early twentieth century when there were some 23,000 funds covering some 14 million workers. Dependents of workers were not covered by sickness funds until the late 1920s. Initially, the employee paid two-thirds, and the employer paid one-third of the contribution. This was later changed to a 50-50 contribution schedule. As Light (1985) points out, Bismarck saw health care as a means of not only increasing the power of the state but also injecting loyalty to the state. Initially, Bismarck wanted a state-run health care system but agreed to the use of sickness funds because of the number of workers already covered through mutual aid societies and the newly emerging sickness funds.

According to Light, Liebfried, and Tennstedt (1986), Bismarck did not get the paternalistic health care system he wanted. Rather, the role of the state became that of "gamemaster and umpire, setting the rules of the system and intervening when it got seriously out of balance" (Light et al. 1986: 78).

Shortly after the passage of the Sickness Insurance Law, the Accident Insurance Law was adopted in 1884, and the Old Age and Invalidity Act in 1889. Built on the following characteristics, these acts were intended to provide low-income workers with limited financial coverage in the event they were unable to continue working.

- Membership in insurance programs is mandated by law for covered workers earning under an income ceiling.
- The administration of these programs is delegated to nonstate bodies governed by representatives of the insured and their employers.
- Entitlement to benefits is linked to past contributions (rather than to other criteria such as need).
- Benefits and contributions are primarily earnings related.
- Financing is secured through wage taxes levied on the employer and the employee and, depending on the program, sometimes by additional financing by the state.
- Until 1997, reimbursement for medical services was made directly to the provider (rather than to the consumer after deduction of copayments, as in France and other neighboring countries). (Altenstetter 1999: 50)

Thus, according to Graig (1999), the German health care system was built on the premise of social solidarity. That is, all citizens should have access to health care, regardless of their ability to pay, and the system is financed through the redistribution of wealth as well as on the basis of age. In other words, "citizens should receive health care benefits according to their needs and should pay according to their ability" (Hoffmeyer 1994: 431). Since its inception, the Sickness Insurance Fund has experienced various reform efforts. However, the basic structure and the resultant benefits have remained largely intact. Even during World War II, when the Nazis controlled the administration of the fund, they did not attempt to limit the basic benefits associated with the system (White 1995).

In addition to solidarity, the principles of subsidiarity and corporatist organization also underlie the German health care system. Subsidiarity refers to a bottom-up approach to the creation of a national health care policy from the sickness funds that were the result of voluntary mutual aid societies. Utilizing this perspective, social organizations thus engage in a public/private power-sharing arrangement. The final principle is that of a corporatist organization. As mentioned earlier, the corporatist arrangement provides for representation of all significant health care players in the decision-making process (Altenstetter 1999).

The foregoing represents the initial period of social insurance in Germany. According to Iglehart (1991a), this period began with the development of social insurance in the mid-1880s to World War I. Subsequent periods include 1915 to 1932, 1933 to 1945, and 1946 to the present (see also Kirkman-Liff 1990 for a timeline of sickness fund/physician relationships). The first period represents the emergence and expansion of sickness funds, and the second period (1915 to 1932) witnessed a shift in the relationship between sickness funds and physicians. Initially, physicians were hired as employees of the sickness funds. By the 1920s, however, many of the funds allowed physicians the decision-making power to divide up the money. This was soon replaced by the development of collective bargaining between physicians' associations and the sickness funds (Schwartz and Busse 1997).

The third period of social insurance begins with the rise to power of Adolf Hitler and ends in 1945. During this period of time, physicians, more than any other profession, joined the National Socialist Party headed by Hitler. The Nazi regime also ousted those physicians considered socialist or non-Aryan. Thus, by the late 1930s, "virtually all physicians sympathetic to autonomous sickness-fund delivery systems had been deported or killed" (Light 1985: 623). Shortly after the end of World War II, Germany became a divided nation with two distinct health care systems. In West Germany, the health care system remained grounded in sickness funds while East Germany constructed a state-run system. The East German system, however, never completely abandoned its roots (Luschen, Niemann, and Apelt 1997). The two health care systems remained until the early 1990s when East and West Germany were reunited after the collapse of the East German communist government.

The state-run East German health care system was constructed on a number of principles that included the following:

- regionally based universal health care
- multitiered provision of care ranging from polyclinics to hospitals

- an emphasis on preventive care and delivery of services at work sites and schools as well as residential locations. (Scharf 1999; see also Ertler et al. 1987; Light 1985)

Briefly, the East German health care system can be characterized as state run and highly centralized. Because health care was funded through payroll and general taxes, services were provided without charge at the point of delivery (Hurst 1991). Examining health outcomes between East and West Germany, the Organization for Economic Cooperation and Development (OECD) (1992) reports that the two countries were similar, although West Germans were healthier. For example, life expectancy in East Germany in 1987 was 69.9 for men and 76.0 for women, whereas it stood at 72.2 for men and 78.9 for women in West Germany. Furthermore, Grosser (1988) points out that infant mortality rates declined from 131.4 to 9.6 by 1985. In addition, mortality rates were similar, regardless of the geographic location, marital status of the mother, or other socioeconomic characteristics. The Organization for Economic Cooperation and Development also points out that whereas West Germany spent 8.5% of GDP on health care, East Germany spent 5.5%. Thus "the former Democratic Republic exhibited a respectable health record for a country with its standard of living" (Organization for Economic Cooperation and Development 1992: 69). Nevertheless, East Germans, particularly males, reportedly were more likely to drink hard liquor, consume more fat, and exercise less than their western counterparts. As a result, East German males experienced considerably higher risks for a variety of diseases (Cockerham 1999).

Health care in West Germany experienced a series of economic crises after World War II. Between 1950 and mid-1970, health care expenditures were increasing at rates ranging from 10% to 20% per year (Schneider 1991). Although the economy had been booming, it fell into recession in the mid-1970s, resulting in a major reform of the health care system. In an effort to control health care costs, a series of Cost Containment Acts were begun in 1977 (Schneider 1994). The initial Cost Containment Act of 1977 was intended to bring "the growth of health care expenditures into line with the growth of wages and salaries of the sickness fund members" (Schneider 1991: 90). In addition, the 1977 act also created a new national level program—the Concerted Action for Health Affairs (CAHA). Consisting of representatives from all affected segments of the health care community as well as officials from all levels of government, CAHA provided recommendations regarding payment increases to health care providers.

In addition to 1977, system-level reforms include the Hospital Cost Containment Act of 1981 and 1982; the Supplementary Cost Containment Act of 1981 and 1982; the Amended Budget Act of 1983; Amended Budget Act of 1984; the Hospital Financing Act of 1985; the Federal Hospital Payment

Regulation of 1986; the Health Care Reform Act of 1989; and the Health Care Structure Reform Act of 1993. More recent reform efforts in the 1990s have attempted to address the increasing costs associated with long-term care. Given space limitations, it is impossible to examine all of these legislative reforms. Therefore, I address the most recent.

The Health Care Structure Reform Act of 1993 was the result of a continued escalation in health care costs and an economic recession. According to Schwartz and Busse (1997), the act was a further attempt to limit growth of health care budgets to that of consumer income. In an effort to achieve its goal, the act placed budget caps on most sectors within the health care community "including hospitals, ambulatory care physicians, prescription pharmaceuticals, and dentists" (U.S. General Accounting Office 1994a: 2). As a result of the act, spending on pharmaceuticals and dentures decreased to 19.6% and 26.9%, respectively, between 1992 and 1993. Although cost increases occurred in other areas, the overall effect was to contain health care costs within the 3% range. Thus, according to Hinrichs (1995), the act has been successful, at least in the short term. The 1993 act also represented "a shift in power from the corporatist institutions toward central government" (Schwartz and Busse 1997: 113).

As mentioned earlier, the 1993 Health Care Reform Act addressed expenditure controls among various components of the health care community. The following overview of these reforms draws extensively from the work of Henke, Murray, and Ade (1994).

The 1993 act limited 1993 physician expenditures to 1991 levels. In future years, expenditure rates were set at the previous year. Dentists, who had commanded higher salaries than physicians, and who had not been subjected to global budgeting in the past, also had expenditure limits placed on them. In an effort to keep physicians and dentists from striking, the law allows for the removal of the person from the sickness fund for upward of six years. Beyond expenditures, the act also attempted to control the volume of services by limiting the number and type (family practitioners rather than specialists) of physicians. Services are limited by monitoring those physicians who provide services at 15% above the average within their specialty area. Physicians who provide services at 25% above the average for their specialty are required to reimburse their association. The 1993 act attempted to control health care costs by "eliminating opportunities for abuse and the potentially negative influence of private profiteering, excessive litigation, and exorbitant claims in malpractice suits" (Stassen 1993: 248).

The 1993 act also limits overall pharmaceutical expenditures as well as the number of prescriptions written by physicians. Setting 24 million DM as the expenditure cap, the act attempts to control the amount of pharmaceuticals being prescribed. Physicians who prescribe 15% over the average are subject to monitoring. If they exceed 25% of the average, they face a reduction in income.

German health care reform efforts have also focused on long-term care. Providing one of the basic foundations of the social insurance system is the Care Insurance Act of 1994. This act is an attempt to address the problems of long-term care for an increasing number of older Germans (Vollmer 2000a, 2000b). The act "provides for extensive nursing home and home-care benefits for peoples of all ages without regard to financial status" (Cuellar and Wiener 2000: 10). Although extensive, the act does not fully cover the cost of long-term care. Individuals remain responsible for approximately 50% of the overall cost of care. Coverage for the act is paid from a premium of 1.7% of a worker's income shared by the employer and employee. In contrast to long-held beliefs in the United States that any new program will exceed initial estimates, the German "program has had an enrollment fairly close to what was initially projected, and expenditures are less than anticipated" (Cuellar and Wiener 1999: 49).

Most recently, health care reform efforts have attempted to address some of the basic weaknesses within the system. Andrea Fischer (1999), the federal minister of health, stated that beginning on January 1, 1999, changes in the system would include reduced co-payments, the coverage of dentures, the elimination of the hospital emergency levy, and other changes. Some of the key components of the Reform Act of SHI (Statutory Health Insurance) 2000 include the following:

- Removal of ineffective or disputed technologies and pharmaceuticals from the sickness funds benefits catalog.
- Improvements in the cooperation of general practitioners, ambulatory specialists, and hospitals.
- Budgets and reimbursement. (European Observatory on Health Care Systems 2000: 115)

The preceding reforms reflect the ongoing changes to the German health care system. Over a hundred years old, the system continues to frame its evolution around those principles that guided its emergence: solidarity, subsidiarity, and a corporatist organization.

## FINANCING AND DELIVERY OF HEALTH CARE

Statutory health insurance funds are financed through work-based contributions from employees and employers. Initially, contribution rates were skewed in favor of employers (one-third) over employees (two-thirds). This ratio was later changed to 50-50 between employees and employers. The contribution is based on wages or salary, rather than the age, sex, or health status of the worker. As a result, there is a redistribution of income to pay for services from the healthy to the poor, the young to the old, and the childless to those with children.

Sickness funds can be divided into two broad categories: state insurance regulation funds and substitute funds. Locally developed state insurance regulation funds provide health care coverage to approximately 40% of the population. Other types of state insurance regulation funds have been developed on the basis of occupation and enterprise. The substitute funds represent the former mutual aid societies that existed when the statutory health insurance scheme was developed. More specifically, there were 453 sickness funds as of June 1, 1999. These funds can be differentiated into these seven distinct groups:

- 17 general regional funds (AOK)
- 13 substitute funds
- 359 company-based funds (BKK)
- 42 guild funds (IKK)
- 20 farmers' funds (LKK)
- 1 miners' fund
- 1 sailors' fund

Depending on the fund, premiums differ. In 1993, for example, the premium for local sickness funds was 14.05%, and the premium for the sailors' fund was 13.10% (Greiner and Schulenburg 1997).

The number of sickness funds decreased throughout the twentieth century. More specifically, the 1990s saw the number of funds decrease from 1,221 in early 1993 to 453 in mid-1999. One reason for the recent decline in the number of sickness funds has been the increased competition for members (Brown and Amelung 1999). Recent reforms allow workers to join any sickness fund they wish. This yearly opportunity has resulted in younger, healthier workers transferring to less expensive funds. As a result, there is increasing concern that the concept of solidarity within the German system may be coming apart.

Currently, 88% of Germans belong to one of the public sickness funds, and 9% have opted out and are covered by private insurance. Another 2% are covered by government health care, and 0.1% are uninsured (European Observatory on Health Care Systems 2000). According to the Organization for Economic Cooperation and Development (1992), the uninsured are individuals who are financially well off. The most current threshold for mandatory participation in the sickness funds is a gross income of $43,466 in the western states and $36,818 in the eastern states (Geraedts, Heller, and Harrington 2000). The average contribution rate is 13.5%. Thus workers and employers each contribute, on average, 6.75% toward coverage.

These are the basic benefits provided by sickness funds:

- Prevention of disease
- Screening for disease
- Treatment of disease (ambulatory medical care, dental care, drugs, nonphysician care, medical devices, inpatient/hospital care, nursing care at home, and certain areas of rehabilitative care)
- Transportation

Other benefits include cash benefits to sick employees. These benefits are initially paid by the sickness fund and later by the government (European Observatory on Health Care Systems 2000).

As mentioned earlier, social insurance now consists of four basic components that consist of health insurance, long-term care insurance, pension insurance, and accident insurance. As of 1997, the average employee/employer percentage contribution within each area was 6.82, 0.85, 3.25, and 10.15, respectively. In the last category, accident insurance, employers contributed an estimated average of 2.50% and employees did not contribute. The average total contribution for employees and employers for all social insurance programs was 21.07% and 23.57%, respectively.

Putting the overall cost of health care in perspective, health care expenditures as a percentage of GDP between 1960 and 1980 were similar to the United States. Per capita health care expenditures, however, have consistently been greater in the United States than Germany. By 1975, Germany spent 8.8% of GDP on health care compared with 8.0% in the United States. After the mid-1980s, health care costs were contained and actually declined between 1985 and 1990. Currently, Germany spends approximately 10.7% of GDP on health care (National Center for Health Statistics 2000). Average annual real growth in per capita health care spending in Germany between 1960 and 1998 increased at 4.2%. The annual rate of growth between 1990 and 1998 was 2.3%. These figures are below the OECD-reported average of 4.5% and 2.4%, respectively, for 23 industrialized nations (see Anderson et al. 2000).

The financing of health care services is primarily through the sickness funds, not the national government. According to the Organization for Economic Cooperation and Development (1992), funding sources include contributions to statutory health insurance (60%), general taxation (21%), private insurance (7%), and out-of-pocket expenses (11%). Negotiations between sickness funds and regional associations determine reimbursement rates for physician and hospital services. According to Schulenburg (1994), 18.2% of sickness fund expenditures go to physicians, 9.7% to dentists, 16.3% for pharmaceuticals, 33.2% for inpatient care, 17.5% for other expenditures/cash payments, and 5.1% for administrative costs. In addition to the sickness funds, a number of private insurance companies exist for those whose incomes are above the threshold as well as those wishing to pay for supplemental services. Within the private health care, sector fees are double what they are in the sickness funds. As Schneider (1994) reports, private health care increased at an annual average of 3.5% compared with 2.5% within the public sector. Although those with private health care coverage receive some institutional perks (private hospital rooms), the overall quality of care is not significantly better than care received through the sickness funds. Furthermore, those who opt out of the sickness funds for private insurance are not allowed to return unless their monthly income falls below the threshold (Schulenburg 1994). Recent efforts (1989–2000) to contain health care costs in ambulatory care, hospitals, and pharmaceuticals have included regulatory features such as fixed budgets and spending caps at all administrative levels (European Observatory on Health Care Systems 2000).

Although the cost of German health care has been increasing, it is instructive to place the system in perspective. Health care in Germany represents one of the most generous systems in the world. Although workers lost one day of vacation as a result of the recent long-term care package, the benefits remain the envy of the industrialized world. Consider the following summation of benefits covered under the German system:

The sickness funds cover the health care costs of both members and their families. They cover ambulatory, hospital, and dental care with little or no copayment. A copayment of an additional DM 11.00 per day for hospital stays has been approved, but unification has delayed its implementation. The bulk of expenditures cover these medical services. In addition, the funds pay for convalescent therapy (cures) and give case benefits to patients, for instance, continued payment for wages during illness grants for young mothers, and reimbursement to patients for eyeglasses and medical appliances. (Schulenburg 1992: 720)

One component that is particularly expensive within the German health care system is pharmaceuticals. This is an area the federal government did not attempt to control until passage of the 1989 Health Care Reform Act (Iglehart 1991b). Although the percentage of the total health care budget consumed by pharmaceuticals and medical devices decreased from 16.2% in 1970 to 12.2% in Germany, by comparison, the United States spent 12.4% and 10.1% of the health care budget on pharmaceuticals and medical devices during the same period of time (Organization for Economic Cooperation and Development 2000). Efforts to control prescription costs through fixed reimbursement process have generally failed because the pharmaceutical industry focused greater emphasis on those drugs not covered in an attempt to make up for profits lost as a result of the reference price listing (Mossialos 1998).

Pharmaceutical costs are greater in Germany than the United States for a number of reasons. First, physicians in Germany are more likely to prescribe medications. According to Schulenburg (1992), German physicians write an average of 11 prescriptions per patient per year. This is some three times the rate of American physicians. Second, reunification of East and West Germany resulted in a substantial increase in the numbers of patients covered through sickness funds that cover most of the cost of prescription drugs on their positive list (Schulenburg 1997). Within a relatively short period of time, former East German consumption of prescription drugs was equivalent to that of West Germans. It took less than two years for former East Berlin to surpass West Berlin in per capita prescription expenditures.

Explanations for the level of growth in pharmaceutical expenditures have focused on sociocultural factors in the east such as a greater likelihood of disease, lower incomes, and lack of employment (Katz 1994). A broader explanation regarding the extensive use of pharmaceuticals in Germany would suggest there is little financial incentive not to request or prescribe medication. Examining the cost of pharmaceuticals in Germany, a U.S. General Accounting Report (1994b) states that prescription drug co-payments range from $1.84 to $4.29. Stated differently, Abel-Smith et al. (1995) indicate that German patients pay 7% of the cost of pharmaceuticals.

Although German health care has experienced efforts for reform, it has weathered attempts to create an American-style system, but recent reforms have introduced increased levels of competition among sickness funds. The remainder of the chapter examines the role of physicians and hospitals as well as the impact of the system on basic sociological variables such as age, sex, social class, and race and ethnicity.

### Physicians

Historically, the relationship between physicians and sickness funds has been contentious (Maynard 1975). The following chronology from Kirkman-Liff (1990) offers insight into the historical relationship between physicians and sickness funds in Germany.

Prior to 1913, a number of payment options existed between physicians and sickness funds. Some were paid on a capitation basis, others were salaried, and others were reimbursed on a fee-for-service basis. With the passage of the Sickness Insurance Act in 1883, reimbursement methods were either capitation or salary. A subsequent 1892 act forbid the use of the fee-for-service option. Resenting these changes, physicians went on strike in 1898. One outcome of the strike was the formation of the Union of German Physicians. Between 1900 and 1911, there were some two hundred strikes per year. Between 1913 and 1933, the relationship between physicians and sickness funds worsened as a result of World War I and the subsequent economic slowdown.

Between 1933 and 1955, the German government provided the means for a fundamental change between physicians and sickness funds. In particular was the creation of physician associations in the early 1930s. Representing the interests of physicians in negotiation with sickness funds, the associations distributed monies from the sickness funds to physicians on a fee-for-service basis. That is, physician services were assigned a point scale and billed to the association based on the point scale. Physicians were then paid from the pool of money collected by the association from the sickness fund.

Between 1955 and 1976, the role of physician associations was further refined as they became centers of claims processing and payment distribution. Physician fee schedules and relative point values of services were established through national negotiations, and payments to physicians differed by region of country.

Further refinement of the relationship between physicians and sickness funds occurred between 1976 and 1986. Perhaps the most significant development during this period was the creation of the Concerted Action in Health Care, an advisory body made up of representatives from all of the major parties in health care. The purpose of the body is articulate government health care policy as well as ensuring that goals established by the government are met. For example, contracts negotiated in 1978 reflected efforts to reduce health care costs by targeting physician expenditures to the previous year, although adjustments could be made given external factors such as population shifts, medical technology, and morbidity.

The final phase extends between 1986 and the present. Kirkman-Liff (1990) argues that expenditure targets identified in the previous time period were not effective in controlling the cost of health care. As a result, the targets were replaced with expenditure caps. In addition, capitated payment rates from sickness funds were linked to wage rate increases of fund members. Revisions in 1987 had the effect of shifting physician fees from "laboratory services to those for personal medical services" (Brenner and Rublee 1991: 155).

Efforts have continued to limit the cost of physician services. One of the outcomes of the 1994 reforms was the implementation of global budgeting of physician expenditures. In addition, the reforms will limit the number of physicians as well as monitor their productivity. Physician organizations have been able to renegotiate fixed budgets and return to fee for service. Given the history of physicians in Germany, it is not surprising that physicians have organized protests against recent reforms. On December 18, 1998, most general practitioners and a large number of specialists staged a one-day strike. They were protesting government efforts to reduce funding for health care (Cooper-Makhorn 1999). In November 1999, some 20,000 physicians were expected to participate in a protest against attempts to reduce health expenditures through the development of a national budget (Durand de Bousingen 1999).

In the last hundred years, physicians in Germany have developed a strong professional presence. As a result, they have remained relatively independent, as demonstrated by their continued location in solo private practice arrangements. As with most European nations, the provision of services between general practitioners and specialists is clearly defined. There is also a clear distinction between office-based and hospital-based physicians. Most office-based physicians do not have hospital-admitting privileges. White (1995) reports that only 12% of hospital beds are for office-based physicians who generally specialize in otolaryngology, pediatrics, and gynecology. Meanwhile, hospital-based physicians are generally on salary. Between 1960 and 1994, physicians have shifted from being office based (62% to 38%) to being hospital based. In 1994, there were more hospital-based physicians (129,100) than office-based physicians (109,300). Furthermore, office-based physicians are increasingly joining group practices rather than maintaining solo practices (Greiner and Schulenburg 1997). Although patients are free to see any doctor, they must receive a referral to see any other doctor besides their primary provider.

Similarly, as in other industrialized nations, the percentage of physicians who are women has been increasing during the past two decades. Currently, approximately 27% of the some 287,000 physicians are women (Lassey, Lassey, and Jinks 1997). At 3.5 physicians per 1,000 persons, Germany has a relatively higher proportion of physicians than most other industrialized nations. According to some estimates, Germany has 25% more physicians than necessary. Nevertheless, problems of physician maldistribution persist. Physicians would evidently remain unemployed than practice in rural areas of the country. Because of recent reform efforts, physician expenditures, the number of services per physician as well as total reimbursement per physician, has been slowed. For example, total reimbursement increased 34% between 1988 and 1992. Between 1992 and 1995, total reimbursement increased by 13%. Reimbursement per physician increased 19% between 1988 and 1992 but declined by 1% between 1992 and 1995. Nevertheless, physician income is approximately three to five times that of blue-collar workers and two to three times that of other white-collar workers (European Observatory in Health Care Systems 2000).

## Hospitals

Historically, hospitals in Germany date to the medieval period where destitute elderly and others unable to care for themselves were housed (see, for example, Stollberg 1993). At the time, hospitals were generally an annex of a church or chapel. By the Middle Ages, hospitals were coming increasingly under the control of the towns within which they were located. Although services were limited, the era of the modern hospital began in the eighteenth century with the separation of patients by disease rather than confining a large number of patients together in the same room. In 1794, hospitals in Prussia were put under state control. Less than a hundred years later, the Social Insurance Act of 1883 included hospital care (Eichhorn 1984).

Today, hospitals in Germany can be categorized into one of three areas of ownership. Local and regional government own 51% of hospitals. Another 35% are under the control of community and church, with the remaining 14% private and for profit (Kirkman-Liff 1999). Hospital ownership arrangements are the result of historical development and regional traditions rather than health policy (Altenstetter 1999). Government-owned and private nonprofit hospitals receive a per diem reimbursement from the sickness funds that covers all services provided by hospital-based salaried physicians. Private for-profit hospitals, which are usually owned by physicians, also receive a per diem reimbursement that does not include payment for physician services (Weil 1992).

Whereas hospital operating revenues are provided by sickness funds, capital expenditures come primarily from state government. These two revenue streams also apply to private for-profit hospitals. All hospitals also negotiate annual global budgets with the sickness funds. These budgets take into account a number of factors such as the current payroll, occupancy rate, and cost of providing services when calculating average daily rates. The fixed-cost break-even volume is also taken into account when determining the average per diem rate. Thus, if actual volume is greater than its break-even volume, "it receives only 25% of the per diem rate for those patient-days in excess of the break-even volume. On the other hand, if the actual volume is less than the break-even volume, then the hospital receives 75% of the per diem rate for those days between its actual volume and the break-even volume" (Kirkman-Liff 1999: 91–92).

Beginning in 1996, case fees and procedure fees were added to a limited number of inpatient areas. Case fees for all patients (except psychiatry) took effect beginning in 2003. Case fees are determined through the combination of diagnosis and intervention. Thus they are similar to diagnostic related groups (DRGs) in the United States. Case fees are generated by determining the cost of a diagnosis among a patient sample minus 15% off the average length of stay among the sample. In contrast, procedure fees address intervention(s).

Although budgets are negotiated between the hospital and sickness funds, they represent targets rather than a specified monetary amount. In addition, case fees have to be reimbursed if hospital activity is above or below the target activity. If hospital activity is above the target, case and procedure fees are reimbursed at 50% or less, depending on the diagnosis and intervention. If hospital activity is below the target, case and proce-dure fees are reimbursed at 40% of the difference (European Observatory on Health Care Systems 2000).

The average length of stay in German hospitals is considerably above that of most OECD countries. In 1998, the average length of stay in German hospitals was 12.0 days. By comparison, the average length of stay in the other five countries presented in this book range from 7.1 days in the United States to 40.8 in Japan (Organization for Economic Cooperation and Development 2000). Excluding Japan, Germany has the longest aver-age length of stay for inpatient care among the countries examined in this book. For an explanation of the Japanese average length of stay, see chap-ter 7.

Explanations for the higher than average length of hospital stay in Ger-many include the distinction between office- and hospital-based physi-cians. As a result, patient information is often not shared, thus requiring duplicate diagnostic procedures when admitted to a hospital. Second, the method of financing hospitalization does not discourage extended stays. Third, most German hospitals do not offer outpatient care (Grogan 1992). With passage of the Health Care Structure Reform Act of 1993, however, the barrier between ambulatory and hospital-based services is slowly breaking down. For example, the 1993 act provides for ambulatory sur-gery departments in hospitals (U.S. General Accounting Office 1994a). The number of inpatient care beds in German hospitals increased from 583,513 in 1960 to 762,596 in 1998. The number of inpatient beds per 1,000 popu-lation, however, declined from 10.5 in 1960 to 9.3 in 1998 (Organization for Economic Cooperation and Development 2000).

Hospital costs are also influenced by the level and extent of medical technology available. In Germany, expensive hospital-based medical tech-nology was not controlled until passage of the Hospital Cost Containment Act in 1982. Acquisition of such technology became part of hospital plan-ning. Between 1989 and 1997, regionally based joint committees that included the hospital and ambulatory sectors became responsible for identifying and controlling expensive medical technology.

The availability of expensive medical technology in German hospitals is increasing. According to the Organization for Economic Cooperation and Development (2000), the number of CT scanners per million population has increased from 5.1 in 1982 to 17.1 in 1997, and MRI devices increased from 1.9 per million in 1990 to 6.2 per million in 1997. Relative to the United States, fewer German hospitals have such technology. Although Rublee (1994) reports fewer medical technologies in Germany than in Canada, a more recent comparison of the percentage of hospitals in the United States, Canada, and Germany with such technology indicates that Canadian hospitals are generally less likely to have expensive medical technology than German hospitals (Weil 1995).

## CURRENT REALITIES AND THE ROLE OF THE STATE

As with other countries, Germany continues to reform its health care system. Reunification of East and West Germany offered an opportunity for political integration, but the cost to the health care system has been significant. Nevertheless, average annual real growth in per capita health spending between 1990 and 1998 increased 2.3% compared to an average of 2.4% in 23 OECD countries (Anderson et al. 2000).

Although Germany has been able to control the cost of health care, gross indicators of the nation's health are of some concern given the level of expenditures on health. For example, 2000 life expectancy rates for males and females (74.3 and 80.8) are mostly lower compared with the United Kingdom (75.0 and 80.5) and Sweden (77.0 and 82.4). Relative to the UK (5.6) and Sweden (3.5), Germany's infant mortality rate (4.8) in 2000 was in the middle (U.S. Bureau of the Census, 2001). However, Germany spent 10.7% of GDP on health care in 1997, and health expenditures as a percentage of GDP in Sweden and the United Kingdom were 8.6 and 6.8%, respectively (National Center for Health Statistics 2000). Furthermore, Greiner and Schulenburg (1997) identify a number of additional problems with the German health care system. One problem is the changing demographic structure of the country. Because most of the revenue for the sickness funds is obtained through wages, continued unemployment and a growing proportion of the population moving into private insurance rather than the statutory insurance program will put pressure on health care funding. A second problem is whether the current level of health care benefits can be maintained.

The European Observatory on Health Care Systems (2000) has raised a similar set of issues that include the following:

- Financing and reimbursement
- Health technology assessment
- Separation between sectors
- Collectivism versus competition

Many of these issues go to the core of the German health care system and reflect the growing influence of a market orientation in health care. As cost control efforts continue to outweigh equality of access, the potential for a multitiered system will become increasingly possible, thus replacing the concept of solidarity with that of self-interest.

The current reality in Germany is that public confidence in their health care system has begun to wane. Germany, like other industrialized nations, is facing difficult choices relative to the primary goals of its health care system. For example, Schulenburg (1992) identifies three goals associated with most health care systems and the difficulty of any system achieving all three. These goals are equal access, competitive pricing, and freedom of choice. Although equal access and freedom of choice characterize the German system, competitive pricing does not. This combination leads to problems of cost control. Germany has implemented some efforts to create competition (i.e., sickness funds competing for members), but the system requires the funds to all provide essentially the same set of benefits.

Given these competing goals, the German health care system has been able to provide quality services with a minimal amount of organizational restructuring. What is apparent in Germany and elsewhere is that supply-side reform efforts have been more successful than have demand-side reforms (Saltman and Figueras 1998).

As evidenced at the beginning of the chapter, the role of the state has been historically prominent in the development and continued refinement of the German health care system. In Germany, there are three levels of government: the federal, the *Lander* (state), and the local. According to Hurst (1991), "the involvement of government in the Western German health system has at least three distinct characteristics:

- A strong legal framework set centrally
- Within this, considerable devolution of power and responsibility to sickness funds, physicians' associations, and other bodies
- Diffusion of the remaining government responsibilities between Federal, State and local governments." (78)

Germany is a federal republic within which 16 states (*Lander*) have adopted their own constitutions. At the federal level, the legislative structure consists of an Assembly with 672 members who are elected every four years. There is also a Federal Council consisting of representatives from the 16 state governments. The Federal Council must approve laws passed by the Assembly. *Landers* have authority to pass laws except in those areas specifically given to the federal government. As a result, there is considerable power sharing between the state and federal governments. Although the federal government creates health policy, approval lies with the state governments. The federal government does not intervene "though it may change by law the regulations governing the statutory requirements of sick funds" (Abel-Smith 1992: 19). State governments:

Supervise negotiations between physicians' associations and sickness funds; take responsibility for hospital planning and investment as well as for managing state-owned hospitals; and regulate medical education, which brings indirect control of the supply of doctors through manipulating the enrolment of medical students. (Freeman 2000: 59)

Nevertheless, the federal government has become increasingly involved in health care through passage of reform laws as well as direct intervention of sickness funds to ensure a redistribution of resources (Harrison and Moran 2000).

In addition to the federal government and the *Lander* is the corporatist level, represented by physicians' associations on the provider side and the sickness funds on the purchaser side (European Observatory on Health Care Systems 2000). The goal of the corporatist level is "to meet the health needs of the population, to provide state-wide services in all medical specialties, and to receive a fixed budget from the sickness funds which the physicians' associations distribute among their members" (Schwartz and Busse 1997: 107).

Although this arrangement raises numerous questions regarding issues such as the organizational structure as well as power differentials within the system, the most intriguing concern involves health outcomes within the population. Given the broad-based concern for national solidarity and therefore health equity, it would be expected that health outcomes would be similar across segments of the population.

## THE HEALTH OF THE POPULATION BY AGE, SEX, SOCIAL CLASS, AND RACE AND ETHNICITY

Similar to the other nations examined throughout this book, the German health care system reflects the social and economic differentiation that exists throughout the larger society. As a result, differential health outcomes persist, despite governmental pronouncement that the health care system is built on equity.

### Age

The German population is becoming increasingly older and smaller. As the death rate exceeds the birthrate, the overall population of the country is expected to decrease. In addition, the percentage of the population aged 65 and over is one of the highest in Western Europe. In 1990, 15% of the population was age 65 and over. By 2010, this segment of the population is expected to reach 20.4% and should increase to 24.4% by 2025. Perhaps more significantly, the percentage of the population aged 80 and over will double from 3.8% in 1990 to 7.7% in 2025 (U.S. Bureau of the Census 1992).

Compared with other industrialized nations, German males and females retire at generally earlier ages. As a result, the percentage of the older age population in the workforce is one of the smallest. In addition, Germany spends a greater percentage of GDP on public pensions than most other industrialized nations and has one of the lowest ratios of population ages 15 to 64 to population age 65 and over. Older individuals in Germany also have one of the highest ratios of income at age 67 compared with their income at age 55 (Anderson and Hussey 2000). Examining explanations for the early retirement of German workers because of disability, Riphahn (1999) argues that the magnitude of unemployment rather than disability benefits has created an incentive for early retirement. A second factor associated with the aging population is that of long-term care. Germany has instituted a long-term care program, but its ability to provide for the increased needs of a rapidly growing population will require continued observation. A third factor influencing the impact of age on health care costs is the use of prescription drugs (see, for example, Freund et al. 2000). Although efforts have been made to reduce the overall cost of pharmaceuticals, an aging society such as Germany can expect increased costs associated with prescription drugs.

Given the availability of social insurance, disability, and long-term care, the cost of providing for the needs of the aging German population continues to increase. Because these programs are primarily structured on a pay-as-you-go method, the potential for economic and social disruption if the economy cannot maintain coverage is an ever-present reality. Further, although the health of the general population has improved (as measured by such gross indicators as life expectancy), it has not achieved the level of other Western European nations. This is also problematic as health care costs continue to increase regardless of age. It is evident that Germany will need to locate a balance between its level of benefits and the ability of the population to pay for them.

### Sex

As with other nations, health differences exist between men and women. These differences, however, are also related to factors such as unemployment, occupation (blue/white collar) and social class position (Kirchgassler 1990; Schwefel 1986). The impact of these economic differences is best illustrated by the fact that earnings by women were, on average, less than one-half (42%) that of the average male wage. Not surprisingly, women constitute almost three-quarters of the welfare caseload in Germany (Lassey and Lassey 2001). Mejer and Siermann (2000) also present evidence of income differences between males and females. They point out that, at all age categories, with the exception of those between 55 and 64, women experience higher poverty rates than men. Not surprisingly, the unemployed (particularly men) experience more health impairments than the employed (Schwefel 1986). Schwefel (1986) also points out that the health status of the unemployed is similar to the employed. In fact, for those in previously strenuous jobs, their health status increased with unemployment.

Men and women also differ regarding age at retirement with women retiring at an earlier age, particularly women enrolled in blue-collar sickness funds. The differences are attributed to the increased levels of physical incapacity associated with occupations covered by blue-collar sickness funds. Although women generally retire earlier than men, mortality and chronic illness rates are generally higher among men than women (Kirchgassler 1990).

### Social Class

Although all Germans have access to health care through a sickness fund or private insurance, health differences on the basis of social class persist. As in other industrialized nations, the higher the social class of Germans, the lower their rates of morbidity and mortality. In addition, Kirchgassler (1990) also provides evidence that workers in white-collar sickness funds continue to experience fewer hospitalization days than members of blue-collar sickness funds. Similarly, blue-collar workers are more likely than white-collar workers to experience chronic illness. Thiede and Traub (1997) offer additional support for the relationship between health and social class when they state that "strong ties exist between a household's income situation and individual health status" (875). Schwefel (1986) provides additional support for the relationship between health and social class.

### Race and Ethnicity

For half a century, the former West Germany has been a magnet for immigrants. By the mid-1990s, Germany was home to some 7 million immigrants primarily from Turkey, the former Yugoslavia, Italy, Greece, and Spain. A breakdown by immigrant ethnic identity can be found in *Facts about Germany* (1997). Although immigrants have provided essential labor in Germany for decades, they remain concentrated in industries associated with higher health risks. Compared with Germans, immigrants were also more likely to be unemployed. Interestingly, immigrants generally report fewer long-term or chronic problems than Germans. However, immigrants, particularly those who are unemployed, are less satisfied with their health status (Elkeles and Seifert 1996).

Access to health care for minorities depends on whether or not they are permanent residents. If permanent, they have access to the same benefits as Germans. However, if they are not permanent residents, only the adult worker has health care benefits. Depending on the income level of the employed adult, other family members are covered either by funds at the county and local level or through their purchase of private insurance (Abel-Smith et al. 1995).

## CONCLUSION

The historical roots of the German health care system lie in a social insurance model characterized by sickness funds. Although Otto von Bismarck originally proposed the creation of a state-run health care system, he agreed to the creation of a national sickness fund for low-wage workers.

The greatest compliment of the German health care system comes from Reinhardt (1994), who states that it "is almost elegant in its simplicity" (23). While Americans continue to debate whether universal health care coverage is possible, Germany has, for over a century, developed a social environment within which the population is accorded the dignity and self-respect associated with being fully actualized members of the society. Through the creation of the Sickness Insurance Act, the Accident Insurance Law, the Old-Age and Invalidity Act, and the more recent Long-Term Care Act, Germany has constructed a foundation of solidarity on which the health care needs of the population are ensured regardless of their age, employment status, or health condition.

The German health care system is currently composed of some 453 sickness funds. Membership in one of these funds is mandatory for all Germans earning below $43,466 as of 1999. Those whose earnings are above this amount have the option of joining a sickness fund or purchasing private health care. The average contribution of sickness fund members is currently 13.5%, with payment coverage divided equally (6.75%) between employee and employer.

Although Germany spends considerably less on health care than the United States, there has been concern regarding growth in the health care sector. Although a market-oriented system such as the United States is unlikely to occur in Germany, sickness funds are becoming interested in the managed care model reminiscent of health maintenance organizations located in the United States. Adaptation of such a model is currently impossible given the freedom of patients to see the physician of their choice (see Jost 1998 for an overview of current issues associated with the German system).

## REFERENCES

Abel-Smith, Brian. 1992. *Cost Containment and New Priorities in Health Care*. Aldershot, UK: Avebury.

Abel-Smith, Brian, Josep Figueras, Walter Holland, Martin Mckee, and Elias Mossialos. 1995. *Choices in Health Policy: An Agenda for the European Union*. Aldershot, UK: Dartmouth.

Altenstetter, Christa. 1999. "From Solidarity to Market Competition? Values, Structure, and Strategy in German Health Policy, 1883–1997." In *Health Care Systems in Transition: An International Perspective,* ed. Francis D. Powell and Albert F. Wessen. Thousand Oaks, CA: Sage.

Anderson, Gerard F., and Peter Sotir Hussey. 2000. "Population Aging: A Comparison among Industrialized Countries." *Health Affairs* 19(3): 191–203.

Anderson, Gerard F., et al. 2000. "Health Spending and Outcomes: Trends in OECD Countries, 1960–1998." *Health Affairs* 19(3): 150–157.

Angus, Douglas E. 1998. "Health Care Costs: Canada in Perspective." In *Health and Canadian Society: Sociological Perspectives,* 3rd ed., ed. David Coburn, Carl D'Arcy, and George Torrance. Toronto: University of Toronto Press.

Blendon, Robert J., Robert Leitman, Ian Morrison, and Karen Donelan. 1990. "Satisfaction with Health Care Systems in Ten Nations." *Health Affairs* 9(2): 185–192.

Blendon, Robert J., John Benson, Karen Donelan, Robert Leitman, Humphrey Taylor, Christian Koeck, and Daniel Gitterman. 1995. "Who Has the Best Health Care System? A Second Look." *Health Affairs* 14(4): 220–230.

Brenner, Gerhard, and Dale A. Rublee. 1991. "The 1987 Revision of Physician Fees in Germany." *Health Affairs* 10(3): 147–156.

Brown, Lawrence D., and Volker E. Amelung. 1999. "'Manacled Competition': Market Reforms in German Health Care." *Health Affairs* 18(3): 76–91.

Cockerham, William C. 1999. *Health and Social Change in Russia and Eastern Europe.* New York: Routledge.

Cooper-Makhorn, Deirdre. 1999. "German Doctors Strike against Health Care Budgets." *British Medical Journal* 318: 78.

Cuellar, Alison Evans, and Joshua M. Wiener. 1999. "Structuring a Universal Long-Term Care Program: The Experience of Germany." *Generations* 23(2): 45–50.

———. 2000. "Can Social Insurance for Long-Term Care Work? The Experience of Germany." *Health Affairs* 19(3): 8–25.

Durand de Bousingen, Denis. 1999. "Doctors Protest against German Health Reforms." *The Lancet* 354: 1103.

Eichhorn, Siegfried. 1984. "Health Services in the Federal Republic of Germany." In *Comparative Health Systems: Descriptive Analyses of Fourteen National Health Systems,* ed. Marshall W. Raffel. University Park: Pennsylvania State University Press.

Elkeles, Thomas, and Wolfgang Seifert. 1996. "Immigrants and Health: Unemployment and Health Risks of Labour Migrants in the Federal Republic of Germany, 1984–1992." *Social Science & Medicine* 43(7): 1035–1047.

Ertler, Wolfgang, H. Schmidt, J. M. Treyth, and H. Wintersberger. 1987. "The Social Dimensions of Health and Health Care: An International Comparison." *Research in the Sociology of Health Care* 5: 1–62.

European Observatory on Health Care Systems. 2000. *Health Care Systems in Transition: Germany.* Copenhagen, Denmark.

*Facts about Germany.* 1997. Frankfort: Press and Information Office of the Federal Government.

Fischer, Andrea. 1999. "A Socially Equitable Health Care Policy." http://www.bmgesundheit.de/engl/health.html. (September 20, 2000).

Freeman, Richard. 2000. *The Politics of Health in Europe*. Manchester, UK: Manchester University Press.

Freund, Deborah A., Don Williams, Grant Reeher, Jarold Cosby, Amy Ferraro, and Bernie O'Brien. 2000. "Outpatient Pharmaceuticals and the Elderly: Policies in Seven Nations." *Health Affairs* 19(3): 259–266.

Geraedts, Max, Geoffrey V. Heller, and Charlene A. Harrington. 2000. "Germany's Long-Term Care Insurance: Putting a Social Insurance Model into Practice." *Milbank Quarterly* 78(3): 375–393.

Graig, Laurene A. 1999. *Health of Nations: An International Perspective on U.S. Health Care Reform*, 3rd ed. Washington, DC: Congressional Quarterly Press.

Greiner, Wolfgang, and J.-Matthias Graf v.d. Schulenburg. 1997. "The Health System of Germany." In *Health Care and Reform in Industrialized Countries*, ed. Marshall W. Raffel. University Park: Pennsylvania State University Press.

Grogan, Colleen M. 1992. "Deciding on Access and Levels of Care: A Comparison of Canada, Britain, Germany and the United States." *Journal of Health Politics, Policy and Law* 17(2): 213–232.

Grosser, Jurgen. 1988. "German Democratic Republic." In *The International Handbook of Health-Care Systems*, ed. Richard B. Saltman. New York: Greenwood Press.

Harrison, Stephen, and Michael Moran. 2000. "Resources and Rationing: Managing Supply and Demand in Health Care." In *Handbook of Social Studies in Health and Medicine*, ed. Gary L. Albrecht, Ray Fitzpatrick, and Susan C. Scrimshaw. Thousand Oaks, CA: Sage.

Henke, Klaus-Dirk, Margaret A. Murray, and Claudia Ade. 1994. "Global Budgeting in Germany: Lessons for the United States." *Health Affairs* 13(4): 5–21.

Hinrichs, Karl. 1995. "The Impact of German Health Insurance Reforms on Redistribution and the Culture of Solidarity." *Journal of Health Politics, Policy and Law* 20(3): 653–687.

Hoffmeyer, Ullrich. 1994. "The Health Care System in Germany." In *Financing Health Care*, Vol. 1, ed. Ullrich K. Hoffmeyer and Thomas R. McCarthy. Dordrecht: Kluwer Academic Publishers.

Hurst, Jeremy W. 1991. "Reform of Health Care in Germany." *Health Care Financing Review* 12(3): 73–86.

Iglehart, John K. 1991a. "Germany's Health Care System. Part 1." *New England Journal of Medicine* 324(7): 503–508.

———. 1991b. "Germany's Health Care System. Part 2." *New England Journal of Medicine* 324(4): 1750–1756.

Jost, Timothy. 1998. "German Health Care Reform: The Next Steps." *Journal of Health Politics, Policy and Law* 23(4): 697–711.

Katz, Eric M. 1994. "Pharmaceutical Spending and German Reunification": Parity Comes Quickly to Berlin." *Health Care Financing Review* 15(3): 141–156.

Kirchgassler, K.-U. 1990. "Health and Social Inequalities in the Federal Republic of Germany." *Social Science & Medicine* 31(3): 249–256.

Kirkman-Liff, Bradford L. 1990. "Physician Payment and Cost-Containment Strategies in West Germany: Suggestions for Medicare Reform." *Journal of Health Politics, Policy and Law* 15(1): 69–99.

————. 1999. "Health Care Cost Containment in Germany." In *Health Care Systems in Transition: An International Perspective,* ed. Francis D. Powell and Albert F. Wessen. Thousand Oaks, CA: Sage.

Lassey, Marie L., William R. Lassey, and Martin J. Jinks. 1997. *Health Care Systems around the World: Characteristics, Issues, Reforms.* Upper Saddle River, NJ: Prentice-Hall.

Lassey, William R., and Marie L. Lassey. 2001. *Quality of Life for Older People: An International Perspective.* Upper Saddle River, NJ: Prentice-Hall.

Light, Donald W. 1985. "Values and Structure in the German Health Care System." *Milbank Memorial Fund Quarterly* 63(4): 615–647.

————. 1997. "Comparative Models of 'Health Care' Systems." In *The Sociology of Health & Illness: Critical Perspectives,* 5th ed., ed. Peter Conrad. New York: St. Martin's.

Light, Donald W., Stephan Liebfried, and Florian Tennstedt. 1986. "Social Medicine vs. Professional Dominance: The German Experience." *American Journal of Public Health* 76: 78–83.

Luschen, Gunther, Steffen Niemann, and Peter Apelt. 1997. "The Integration of Two Health Systems: Social Stratification, Work and Health in East and West Germany." *Social Science and Medicine* 44(6): 883–899.

Lynch, Matthew J., and Stanley S. Raphael. 1963. *Medicine and the State.* Springfield, IL: Charles C. Thomas.

Maynard, Alan. 1975. *Health Care in the European Community.* Pittsburgh: University of Pittsburgh Press.

Mejer, Lene, and Clemens Siermann. 2000. "Income Poverty in the European Union: Children, Gender and Poverty gaps." Themes 3–12/2000. Population and Social Conditions. *Statistics in Focus.* Eurostat. European Union. www.europa.eu.int. (March 20, 2000).

Mossialos, Elias. 1998. "Regulating Expenditure on Medicines in European Union Countries." In *Critical Challenges for Health Care Reform in Europe,* ed. Richard B. Saltman, Josep Figueras, and Constantino Sakellarides. Buckingham, UK: Open University Press.

National Center for Health Statistics. 2000. *Health United States, 2000.* Washington, DC: U.S. Government Printing Office.

Organization for Economic Cooperation and Development. 1992. *The Reform of Health Care: A Comparative Analysis of Seven OECD Countries.* Health Policy Studies No. 2. Paris, France.

————. 2000. *OECD Health Data 2000: A Comparative Analysis of 29 Countries.* Paris, France.

Pfaff, Martin, and Dietmar Wassener. 2000. "Germany." *Journal of Health Politics, Policy and Law* 25(5): 907–914.

Reinhardt, Uwe. E. 1994. "Germany's Health Care System: It's Not the American Way." *Health Affairs* 13(4): 22–24.

Riphahn, R.T. 1999. "Disability Retirement among German Men in the 1980s." *Industrial and Labor Relations Review* 52(4): 628–647.

Roemer, Milton I. 1991. *The Countries.* Vol. 1 of *National Health Systems of the World.* New York: Oxford.

Rublee, Dale A. 1994. "Medical Technology in Canada, Germany, and the United States: An Update." *Health Affairs* 13(4): 113–117.

Saltman, Richard B., and Josep Figueras. 1998. "Analyzing the Evidence on European Health Care Reforms." *Health Affairs* 17(2): 85–108.

Scharf, Bradley. 1999. "German Unity and Health Care Reform." In *Health Care Systems in Transition: An International Perspective,* ed. Francis D. Powell and Albert F. Wessen. Thousand Oaks, CA: Sage.

Schneider, Markus. 1991. "Health Care Cost Containment in the Federal Republic of Germany." *Health Care Financing Review* 12(3): 87–101.

———. 1994. "Evaluation of Cost-Containment Acts in Germany." *Health: Quality and Choice.* Health Policy Studies, No. 4. Organization for Economic Cooperation and Development. Paris, France.

Schulenburg, J.-Matthias Graf von der. 1992. "The German Health Care System: Concurrent Solidarity, Freedom of Choice, and Cost Control." In *Health Care Systems and Their Patients: An International Perspective,* ed. Marilynn M. Rosenthal and Marcel Frenkel. Boulder, CO: Westview Press.

———. 1994. "Forming and Reforming the Market for Third-Party Purchasing of Health Care: A German Perspective." *Social Science & Medicine* 39(10): 1473–1481.

———. 1997. "Economic Evaluation of Medical Technologies: From Theory to Practice—The German Perspective." *Social Science & Medicine* 45(4): 621–633.

Schwartz, Friedrich Wilhelm, and Reinhard Busse. 1997. "Germany." In *Health Care Reform: Learning from International Experience,* ed. Chris Ham. Buckingham, UK: Open University Press.

Schwefel, Detlef. 1986. "Unemployment, Health and Health Services in German-Speaking Countries." *Social Science & Medicine* 22(4): 409–430.

Stassen, Manfred. 1993. "The German Statutory Health Insurance System." *Social Education* 57(5): 247–248.

Stollberg, Gunnar. 1993. "Health and Illness in German Workers' Autobiographies from the Nineteenth and Early Twentieth Centuries." *Social History of Medicine* 6(2): 261–276.

Thiede, Michael, and Stefan Traub. 1997. "Mutual Influences of Health and Poverty. Evidence from German Panel Data." *Social Science & Medicine* 45(6): 867–877.

U.S. Bureau of the Census. 1992. International Population Reports, P25, 92–3, *An Aging World II.* Washington, DC: Government Printing Office.

———. 2001. International Program Center. International Data Base. Washington, DC: Government Printing Office.

U.S. General Accounting Office. 1994a. *German Health Reforms: Changes Result in Lower Health Care Costs in 1993.* (GAO/HEHS-95-27, December). Washington, DC: Government Printing Office.

———. 1994b. *Prescription Drugs: Spending Controls in Four European Countries.* (GAO/HEHS-94-30). Washington, DC: Government Printing Office.

Vollmer, Rudolf J. 2000a. "Long-Term Care Insurance in Germany." Paper presented at the European Seminar on Dependency: A New Challenge for Social Protection. Porto, May 11–14, 2000. http://www.bmgesundheit.de/engl/portugal.html. (March 15, 2001).

———. 2000b. "Long-Term Care Insurance in Germany. Background Paper: Including Issues Related to Dementia and the Quality of Care." Prepared for the Meeting of the OECD Workshop "Healthy Aging and Biotechnology" in Tokyo, Japan, November 13–14, 2000. http://www.bmgesudheit.de (March 15, 2001).

Weil, Thomas P. 1992. "The German Health Care System: A Model for Hospital Reform in the United States?" *Hospital & Hospital Services Administration* 37(4): 533–547.

———. 1995. "Comparisons of Medical Technology in Canadian, German and U.S. Hospitals." *Hospital & Health Services Administration* 40(4): 524–533.

White, Joseph. 1995. *Competing Solutions: American Health Care Proposals and International Experience.* Washington, DC: The Brookings Institution.

World Health Organization. 2000. *World Health Report 2000. Health Systems: Improving Performance.* Geneva, Switzerland.

# CHAPTER 6

# Sweden

The Swedish (or Nordic) model in social policy is *inter alia* characterized by *public* responsibility; comprehensiveness (in respect of *both* covering the whole population *and* including a wide range of services; and solidarity. The idea of general welfare, not only assisting the poor but giving a basic security to everyone, is that the social system shall be financially supported by all and that the quality shall be of a high and even standard. Social services are mainly financed by taxes.

(Bergman 1998: 92)

## INTRODUCTION

The Swedish health care system represents what is perhaps the most comprehensive effort to integrate the economic and social needs of a population. In addition to universal health care coverage, the national health insurance program covers work-related accidents, pension care, and unemployment. Thus, in addition to the in-kind benefit payments made at the county level, cash benefits representing at least 75% of income, "public services for health care; and social care for children, the elderly, and the disabled" (Diderichsen 2000: 931) are also provided. More specifically, these cash benefits include an increasing percentage of income paid to workers the longer they are ill. Parental benefits begin two months prior to the birth of a child and last until the child is 8 years old. Within that time frame, parents can receive benefits for 450 days. The sickness and parental benefits are taxable income. Maternity benefits are also available to women unable to work because of pregnancy. This benefit is equivalent to the parental benefit and can be received for a maximum of 50 days prior to childbirth. Finally, cash benefits also cover additional expenses such as transportation, medicine, and other medical expenses (Hoffmeyer 1994).

Angus (1998) locates the Swedish system in the Beveridge model, indicating universal health care coverage and financed primarily through general taxes. Similarities with the National Health Service in the United Kingdom are particularly evident (Ham, 1988). As Anderson (1972) points out, "enrollment in government-sponsored health insurance is mandatory for the total population" (7). Health care in Sweden is regionally based, although health care is organized at the national, regional, and local levels (World Health Organization 1996).

For years, the Swedish health care system has been the envy of the industrialized world because of its universal coverage and improving indicators of health (see, for example, Lindbeck 1997 for an analysis of the Swedish experiment). Nevertheless, the cost of health care in Sweden has been an area of concern. However, "when current expenditure figures are age adjusted, the Swedish system is only half as expensive as the U.S. system on a per capita basis" (Saltman 1990: 599). The ability of Sweden to provide health care coverage for all and simultaneously control the overall cost of health care reflects the country's commitment to a social democratic philosophy (Andrain 1998).

Currently, the World Health Organization (2000) ranks the Swedish system 23rd in the world in overall performance. Life expectancy rates for males and females were 77.1 and 81.9, respectively (WHO 2000). Sweden is also unique relative to other industrialized nations in that health care costs have been contained throughout the 1990s. For example, Sweden was spending 8.8% of GDP on health care expenditures in 1990, but only 8.6% in 1998. Similarly, per capita spending also decreased from $1,861 in 1990 to $1,820 in 1998 (Anderson et al. 2000). Interestingly, in 1960, the United States and Sweden were spending a similar percentage of GDP on health care. By 1970, Sweden was spending a greater percentage of GDP than the United States. However, since 1980, health care expenditures in the United States have continued to increase, whereas Sweden has been able to control its health care expenditures (Organization for Economic Cooperation and Development 2000).

Although somewhat dated, research indicates that Swedes are less satisfied with their health care system than are Canadians and West Germans. Blendon et al. (1990) report that 32% of Swedes believe their health care system needs only minor changes; 58% stated that fundamental changes were needed; and 6% argued for a complete rebuilding of the system. By comparison, 56% of Canadians and 41% of West Germans felt their health care systems needed only minor change. Furthermore, 38% of Canadians and 35% of West Germans believed fundamental change was needed. Finally, 5% of Canadians and 13% of West Germans believed the health care system needed to be completely rebuilt. Further research efforts support these findings. According to the Organization for Economic Cooperation and Development (2000), public satisfaction with the health care system indicate that in Sweden, 67.3% were very or fairly satisfied, whereas 16.7% were neither satisfied nor dissatisfied and 14.2% were very or fairly dissatisfied. By comparison, the responses in Germany were 66%, 21.4%, and 10.9%, respectively. Stated somewhat differently, 28.5% believe the system runs quite well. Furthermore, 44.1% stated that minor changes are needed and 21.8% agreed that fundamental changes are needed. Finally, 3.4% of respondents in Sweden agreed the health care system should be completely rebuilt. Again, by comparison, the responses in Germany were 36.9%, 38.5%, 16.7%, and 2.2%, respectively.

The need for change within the Swedish health care system is the result of numerous problems. For example, because of an increasingly aged population, there is a growing demand for health care. An interconnected problem is the increased utilization of medical technologies that improve diagnosis and treatment of diseases. In addition to utilization, there has also been extensive growth in the number of such services available within the medical community. An economic reason for possible change within the Swedish health care system is the level of public expenditure on health and social services. Currently, one-third of Sweden's GDP is spent on the public sector. Additional growth in this sector is generally viewed as impossible. Furthermore, the number of health care personnel has increased significantly. Currently, health care personnel constitute over 11% of the total labor force in Sweden.

As mentioned earlier, there is growing discontent among Swedes regarding the level and quality of health care services provided. However, not all concern has focused on economic issues. For example, Ostman (1992) has reservations regarding efforts to create a more effective system because such "an eagerness to economize will lead our public medical care system into a period of stagnation" (199). Finally, economic constraints on the Swedish health care system will necessitate the need for greater efficiency and productivity within the system (Wennstrom 1992).

## HISTORY OF THE SWEDISH HEALTH CARE SYSTEM

Historically, health care in Sweden dates to the ninth century with the arrival of Christian monks (Borgenhammer 1984). The financing of health care emerged during the Middle Ages with the development of community coin chests. These coin chests were the forerunner of medieval guilds that later became provident societies. Although a chair of surgery was created in Uppsala in 1595, there was little effort to expand medical care on a national level (Lynch and Raphael 1963). Throughout this period, the church was primarily responsible for providing medical care at the local level (Wennstrom 1992).

By the seventeenth century, however, community-financed physicians were providing care throughout the country. The first hospital in Sweden was constructed in 1752. Shortly thereafter, the Diet of the Four Estates provided for the creation of hospitals funded through resources collected at the community level. This represented the beginning of a publicly funded health care system in the country with responsibility located at the national level. Historically, the supervision of health services has been the responsibility of various organizations. Currently, that responsibility lies with the National Board of Health and Welfare. The provision of health care is the responsibility of the 23 county councils and 3 large municipalities.

Created in 1862, county councils represent another governmental level that has the power to raise taxes (World Health Organization 1996). Two years later, the operation of hospitals in Sweden was turned over to the county councils (Saltman 1988). The transition of health care responsibility from the central government to county councils occurred over an extended period of time. According to Lassey, Lassey, and Jinks (1997), citizens in Sweden have had virtually free access to health care since 1900 when a tax on liquor was converted to a personal property and income tax intended to pay for health care. However, even with passage of the Sickness Fund Laws of 1891 and 1910 in which government subsidies provided cash subsidies covering lost wages, a relatively small percentage of workers were covered. Anderson (1972) reports that only 13.4% of the adult population were members of sickness funds in 1910. Membership in sickness funds did not increase during the early twentieth century; Immergut (1999) also found that less than 14% of the population was enrolled in sickness funds in 1925. Throughout the early twentieth century, sickness funds emerged as the primary vehicle for insuring workers against the cost of medical care. The federal government also increased its regulatory powers over sickness funds. For example, an 1891 law required state registration by all sickness funds.

By 1931, the state limited the number of sickness funds that could operate within a geographical region. The state also established a minimum level of benefits to be offered by sickness funds and required them to provide open membership (Lynch and Raphael 1963).

The 1928 Hospital Act mandated that county councils were responsible for hospital care of their residents. Additional reform efforts include the 1931 Sickness Funds Act. This act provided state monies to approved health insurance funds (Freeman 2000). In the 1930s, county councils assumed responsibility for nonhospital services. By the 1950s, county councils were providing outpatient care and by 1967, mental health care. The most important legislative act during this period of time was the National Health Insurance Act of 1946. Implemented in 1955, the act was the beginning of universal health care in Sweden. As a result of this act, a national health insurance system was implemented and financed by contributions from the state and employers. The implementation of a compulsory health care system utilized existing public sickness funds. These funds "were independent corporate organizations with financial responsibility for their own activities" (Lynch and Raphael 1963: 269). Although Sweden created a universal health care system, the 1948 Hojer proposal would have established a national health service in Sweden similar to the United Kingdom. For example, the Hojer proposal would have consolidated "all forms of outpatient care into one system under the auspices of the County Councils and the eventual transfer of all doctors to full-time salaries" (Immergut 1992: 205). The Swedish Medical Association adamantly opposed the proposal and lobbied throughout the media against the proposal and its author. Additional system changes during this period include the development of a regional hospital system in 1958 and the elimination of fee for service and private beds for hospital physicians in 1959.

In 1960, outpatient care became the responsibility of county councils. Throughout the 1960s, responsibility for district medical officers and mental hospitals was also transferred to county councils. Passage of the 7-crown reform in 1970 required patients to pay 7 crowns to the county council for each outpatient visit. The reform also located responsibility for outpatient hospital services with the county councils. In 1971, Sweden nationalized the retail distribution of pharmaceuticals. By 1983, all health service planning was transferred to the county councils (see Freeman 2000 for a timeline of significant health reform efforts in Sweden).

Given the extent of health care reform efforts throughout the previous two centuries, Saltman (1988) argues that the most important policy development in Swedish health care has been the development of an emphasis on primary care and an effort to remove those barriers that deny equal access to health care services. Health care in Sweden is thus considered a basic human right that impacts on other individual rights (Whitehead 1998). Reinforcing the responsibility of county councils and the provision of health services was the Dagmar Reform of 1985. The Federation of County Councils (1990) also identifies a number of innovative programs at the county council level. Additional health care reform efforts throughout the early 1990s include an increased emphasis on internal markets (1991–1994), family doctor reform (1994), free establishment of doctors (1994), a maximum waiting time guarantee (1992), and the care of the elderly (1992) (Rehnberg 1997). The movement toward an internal market emphasized the need to separate "the purchaser and provider roles within the county councils" (Rehnberg 1997: 68–69). However, only one-third of county councils representing 40% of the population had done so by 1994.

According to Rehnberg (1997), an internal market in Sweden is based on the following characteristics:

- Collective purchasing units
- Freedom of choice for consumers
- Provider competition
- Contracts and performance-based reimbursement
- Provider autonomy. (69)

The family doctor reform was an effort to give patients a choice in selecting a family physician. Created under the auspices of a conservative government, and without consultation from the medical community, the free establishment for private practitioners reform allowed private practitioners to establish private practices without permission from the county councils. When the Family Doctor Act was proposed, many of the physicians in Sweden went on strike (Freeman and Moran 2000). With the return of a socialist government, this reform was eliminated. The maximum waiting time guarantee was an effort to reduce the length of time patients were required to wait for certain services. If the specific service could not be performed within three months, the patient would be referred to another hospital, a private hospital, or a hospital out of the country. The result is increased efficiency and shorter waiting periods. Finally, the care of the elderly reform transferred long-term care beds from county councils to municipalities. In addition, municipalities also became financially responsible for those patients discharged from hospitals. The reforms of the early to mid-1990s have, for the most part, been negated by the reemergence of the Social Democrats to power at the county and national levels. Although some of the competitive reforms remain (Patient Choice and the Care Guarantee), most others had not proven effective. For example, Harrison and Calltrop (2000) argue, "that purchaser-provider splits—which were only implemented in a minority of counties—played a small role in enhancing productivity" (226). Instead, Harrison and Calltrop contend that budget cuts were far more effective in improving hospital performance.

More recently, health care reform since 1998 has attempted to focus on a number of goals that include efforts

- To foster promotive and preventive activities; both within and outside the health sector;
- To secure equal access to health services of high quality; also for people living in sparsely populated areas;
- To enhance the shift from inpatient hospital care to outpatient care. (Bergman 1998: 93)

Perhaps the most interesting outcome of these recent reform efforts is the lack of overall support for increased privatization of health care. Furthermore, any attempt to reform the system is generally tested first on a small scale at the county or municipal levels before being instituted on a national level (Bergman 1998). Because the Swedish system is decentralized, local officials and county residents are all stakeholders in the health care system. Thus the approach ensures incremental rather than sweeping national reform outcomes (Rathwell 1998). Although devolution is considered a positive influence on the overall provision of health care, it is not without criticism. Diderichsen (1999) argues that as cost control measures are implemented, providers are moving into the private sector. As a result, efforts to control "a growing private sector will need national legislation, but that, in turn, will limit the freedom of local government" (Diderichsen 1999: 1157). More recently, some county councils have begun efforts to merge, thus creating a regionalized health service.

## FINANCING AND DELIVERY OF HEALTH CARE

Health care in Sweden ensures universal access regardless of a person's geographic location or social status. The Swedish health care system is financed primarily through taxation at the county level. In turn, the majority of county expenditures are for health care costs. Health care in Sweden represents a combination of characteristics with a financing scheme similar to the United Kingdom's (see, for example, Saltman and Figueras 1998). Health care financing at the country level comes primarily from tax revenues (72%) with additional monies from the central government (11.2%), out-of pocket expenses (3.5%), and reimbursements from other localities for the provision of health care to their residents (6.2%). All employers contribute 5.28% of a worker's salary to fund the health care system (World Health Organization 1996). More specifically, the 1990 average payroll tax at the county level is 14%, with a range of 12.75% to 14.5%. The average municipal tax rate was 17.3%, with a range of 11.4% to 18.0% (Hoffmeyer 1994).

Organizationally, the Swedish health care system is similar to Canada's. In other words, there are 26 independent health care systems (23 county councils and 3 municipalities) in Sweden. All of these systems "can determine the administrative means by which they will seek to achieve nationally established health policy objectives" (Saltman 1991: 616). The 23 county councils and 3 municipalities provide services in 9 regional hospitals, 84 county/district hospitals, and some 950 health centers throughout the country. At the local level there are 288 municipalities with local control over institutional housing and facilities for the aging and disabled populations (World Health Organization 1996). In addition, Sweden maintains health centers specifically for the needs of children. These centers provide immunization and hearing, vision, and speech screening (Chaulk, 1994). Support for the public health care system and the myriad social programs available to all citizens are financed by the highest taxation rate in the industrialized world. Currently, 50% of income is paid in the form of taxes (Lassey and Lassey 2001). Bjorkman (1985) suggests that the responsibility for ensuring health care to all residents is similar to regional health authorities in England.

Previously, health care institutions and salaried staff, including physicians, received a global budget from the county council. This budget represented the extent and range of services provided in the previous year as well as salaries for staff, including physicians. Although this approach ensured macroeconomic discipline, it was considered less successful at creating microeconomic efficiency (Saltman 1992). As a result of increased waiting times for some medical procedures such as hip replacement, new methods of health care financing at the county level have been implemented. For example, in 1992, the Stockholm county council implemented a planned market experiment referred to as the Stockholm model. Essentially, hospital services are financed creating internal markets in which local health districts purchase hospital services for their patients. This agreement is renegotiated annually between the local health districts and the hospitals. Included in the negotiation is "the scope of service, price, quality, availability, and channels of cooperation among health care providers" (Organization for Economic Cooperation and Development 1994: 279). Over time, hospitals are expected to become financially self-sufficient. In addition, hospitals are implementing the use of diagnostic related groups (DRGs) as a measure of patient care (see also Saltman 1995).

A second financing reform model in Sweden is the Dalamodel. Implemented in a rural county, the Dalamodel distributes "prospectively set hospital budgets to local primary health care boards" (von Otto 1999: 271). The expected outcome of this reform effort is to create incentives "for the primary care centers attached to these local boards to reduce their rate of hospital referrals, and to monitor the necessity of specialist services provided to referred patients" (Saltman 1991: 618). Although these reforms have attempted to instill a market philosophy within the Swedish health care system, it is important to note that hospitals and health centers were not privatized (Saltman 1999).

In addition to the public system, a small but growing private health care sector has emerged in Sweden. As of 1996, private health insurance accounted for 2% of total health care expenditures. Private insurance generally provides supplemental coverage for those services not provided by the national social insurance program (World Health Organization 1996). In 1990, about 15,000 private insurance policies had been issued. The inability to claim private insurance policies as a tax deduction has been cited as one of the reasons for the limited number of policies (Organization for Economic Cooperation and Development 1994). Utilization of private health care also differs by geographic region and age. For example, governments have increasingly employed private health care providers for elder care. Also, utilization rates of private health providers are higher in urban rather than rural areas (Hakansson and Nordling 1997). Interestingly, von Otto (1999) argues that the implementation of some market principles within the health care system has not significantly controlled costs as effectively as some nonmarket reforms. Nevertheless, physicians in the private sector now account for 20% of all consultations (Andersen, Smedby, and Vagero 1997).

### Physicians

Historically, the state has been actively involved in decisions regarding medical practice. In fact, the level of government involvement in Sweden has been identified as one reason why physicians have not pursued greater professional control over their craft. For example, physicians in Sweden during the seventeenth and eighteenth centuries "acted more like public officials than representatives of a free and independent profession" (Garpenby 1999: 410). Although professional organizations for physicians were established in the nineteenth and twentieth centuries (the Swedish Society of Medicine and the Swedish Medical Association, respectively), the power of physicians lies primarily with their specialty organizations (see also Freeman 2000). The level of government involvement in the medical profession is also illustrated by the fact that physicians in Sweden have been employees of the state. In the latter 1800s, the government employed 90% of the physicians. By the 1970s, the percentage of physicians employed by the government had dropped to around 66% (Riska 1993). According to the World Health Organization (1996), however, 89% of physicians are employed in primary health care centers and are paid a salary. Beginning in the 1990s, the government of Sweden initiated the Stockholm model, which has attempted to move physicians into private practice where they would compete for patients. The emergence of this model has fundamentally altered not only how physicians practice medicine, but also their method of reimbursement. Previously, physicians were paid a monthly salary by the government. Under the Stockholm model, physicians would be reimbursed through a capitation system. According to Quaye (1997), physician responses to the Stockholm model vary. On the one hand, physicians report that the model has improved productivity, decreased waiting lists, and has improved the attitude of caregivers. On the other, physicians also reported that the use of DRGs by the Stockholm model could lead to increased utilization of high-cost procedures. Many physicians also suggested that the quality of patient care could suffer, particularly for elderly patients.

Medical training in Sweden occurs in a number of universities throughout the country. The 900 students admitted to medical school yearly are required to complete a 5.5-year program of study and an 18-month pre-registration period as a house officer. Although authorized to practice medicine after this period of training, most doctors continue for an additional 5 years of study in one of the 62 specialty areas (Swedish Institute 1999a). Physicians then request permission to practice medicine from county councils, which make appointments based on need.

Medical practice in Sweden generally occurs within three categories: district medical officers, hospitals, and private practice. Ranking physicians by status, Lassey et al. (1997) locate those in internships or specialist training at the bottom followed by specialists providing outpatient or inpatient services in hospitals. District physicians and heads of clinical hospital units are accorded the next highest status. The highest status for a physician is in an administrative capacity as head of a facility.

Compared with other industrialized nations, Sweden has a relatively high percentage of physicians in specialty areas. According to the Organization for Economic Cooperation and Development (2000), Sweden has a higher ratio of practicing specialists (2.2) and practicing physicians (3.1) per 1,000 population than the United States (1.4 and 2.6, respectively). Among the other countries examined here, only Germany is comparable at 2.1 practicing specialists per 1,000 population. In contrast, Canada has 0.9 practicing specialists per 1,000 population. Sweden has fewer practicing physicians per 1,000 population (3.1) than Germany (3.4) but more than Canada (2.1), Japan (1.8), and the United Kingdom (1.6).

Although most physicians in Sweden are employed by the state, they are poorly distributed throughout the country. As a result, rural areas of Sweden continue to experience problems attracting and retaining physicians. At the same time, Sweden experienced problems of finding positions for all practicing physicians. Although a surplus of physicians was noted in the mid-1990s, there is concern that the country may experience a shortage in the near future. Currently, some 100 physicians are receiving unemployment benefits and 600 registered with the national unemployment bureaus are seeking jobs (Swedish Medical Association 2000).

### Hospitals

Historically, hospitals in Sweden have been public institutions. In addition, a chronic shortage of physicians and other health care personnel throughout the twentieth century forced most medical care into the hospital environment. As a result, the number of available hospital beds and attendant personnel has been extensive and has impacted the overall cost of health care. When Axel Hojer, director general of the National Board of Health and Welfare, in 1948 attempted to increase the number of health centers, he was replaced in 1952 by a director general who was more hospital oriented. At the same time, there was a surge in hospital construction in Sweden (Borgenhammer 1984). Throughout the 1990s, however, the number of available hospital beds and their rate per 1,000 population decreased. This is the result of "increases in productivity generated by new medical technology, shrinking financial resources, and incentives resulting from the development of financial management systems" (Hakansson and Nordling 1997: 196). An example of the change in financial management is the effort within hospitals to provide patients with a limited waiting period for services. If the waiting period exceeds the guaranteed time frame, the patient can secure treatment elsewhere. Previously, hospitals were provided annual global budgets from which they provided services and paid staff, including physicians. Recent reforms, however, have altered that relationship to allow health care funds to follow the patient (see, for example, Wiley 1994).

Hospitals in Sweden consist primarily of three types: general acute, psychiatric, and long-term care (Lassey et al. 1997), and the following illustrates their organization by size (number of beds), level of specialization, and size of population served.

1. At the regional level a single regional hospital serves a population of a million or more. The superspecialties are concentrated at this level.

2. The county central hospital serves a population from 250,000 to 300,000. As a rule this hospital has 800 to 1,000 beds, most of the usual specialties, a large outpatient department, rehabilitation facilities, family planning, welfare services, etc.

3. The local district hospital, typically serving 60,000 to 90,000, is still in the process of transition. Nearly all authorities agree on the need for merging, closing, or converting many of the formerly small district hospitals into nursing homes, health centers, or a combination of the two. Local resistance is considerable, but the policy remains to eliminate all district hospitals with less than 300 beds.

4. The local health center, serving a population of 10,000 to 20,000 with ambulatory preventive and curative care, is not formally part of the hospital system. However, with 300 such centers in operation today, the goal is to integrate their activities with the nearest district hospital. (Somers and Somers 1977: 371; see also Roemer 1991)

This arrangement represents an effort toward a rational configuration of health care facilities throughout the country. However, the cost of delivering health services through a regionalized hospital system has been expensive. As a result, efforts to limit health care costs have included the closing of hospitals and reducing the number of health care personnel.

Compared with most industrialized nations, Sweden has more medical technology per million population than most other European nations. Canada and the United Kingdom have fewer units per million population; the number of units in Germany is similar to Sweden's. The United States and Japan have considerably higher numbers of MRIs and CT scanners per million population (Organization for Economic Cooperation and Development 2000). Although medical technology provides the health care community with a powerful weapon in the diagnosis and treatment of disease, it is, nevertheless, an expensive component of the health care system.

In addition to medical technology, pharmaceuticals also represent a potentially expensive, yet efficient, tool in treating disease. Pharmaceutical expenditures as a percentage of GDP as well as per capita locate Sweden below average compared with other OECD countries (Henriksson, Hjortsberg, and Rehnberg 1999). Nevertheless, pharmaceuticals represent an increasing expenditure within the Swedish health care system. In the early 1990s, Sweden instituted a reference price system that initially contained the cost of pharmaceuticals. Under the program, the national health insurance system will pay the reference price that is determined by its generic equivalent plus 10% (General Accounting Office 1994). However, prices continued to increase after the first year (Mossialos 1998). A more recent effort to control rising prices is a 1998 pharmaceutical reform measure giving county councils financial responsibility for prescriptions. It is expected that the incentives that have controlled the costs of pharmaceuticals in hospitals will be applied to ambulatory and prescription drugs as well. However, there is considerable concern regarding how prescription drugs will be dispensed and the increasing use of patient copayments (Nilsson 1997). Efforts to increase the accessibility of new drugs to patients have come under scrutiny, not only in Sweden, but also throughout Europe. Sweden has been particularly concerned over attempts to decrease the time limits for drug approval. The reason for increased concern in Sweden is attributed to "a regulatory culture which is more sensitive to the public interest" (Abraham and Lewis 1999: 1665).

As the preceding section has demonstrated, health care in Sweden has attempted to maintain the principles of equity and solidarity. However, according to Anderson et al. (1997), Sweden is experiencing a dilemma: maintain health care coverage for all or impose limitations on spending and delivery of health care services.

## CURRENT REALITIES AND ROLE OF THE STATE

Politically, there are three levels of government in Sweden: central, county, and local. Relative to health care, the central government creates those laws on which the health care system is based. According to the

Swedish Institute (1999a), the most important of these laws was the Health and Medical Services Act of 1982 because it established universal access and equality of services. A number of agencies within the central government are responsible for specific aspects of the health care system. The function of the Ministry of Health and Social Affairs is to develop new legislation and government regulations. The National Board of Health and Welfare functions as an advisory and supervisory body. It determines if the provision of government services is consistent with their legislative intent. In addition to setting national policy, the central government is also responsible for accrediting those in the medical field as well as the facilities within which they work. Third, the national government is responsible for medical malpractice and discipline. A fourth responsibility of the national government is that of special grants and payments. In other words, the national government will compensate those counties that have a below-average tax base to ensure equal access to all citizens, regardless of where they live. The national government also provides economic support for teaching and research at university hospitals. Fifth, the national government has established a technology evaluation center. The purpose of the center is to establish uses for new technology. Finally, because the national government funds medical education, it also determines the number of students, curriculum, as well as overall size of the medical profession (Saltman 1999).

Although the central government creates the legislation and regulations defining how health care will be provided, county councils are responsible for financing and implementing these services. County councils have been overseeing a number of fundamental reforms within the Swedish health care system. For example, patients are now free to choose their health care provider even if the person is outside the county in which the patient resides.

The local level of government is primarily responsible for the elderly and disabled. Local officials also have responsibility to cover the cost of care for those patients remaining in hospital if alternative residential options such as a nursing home bed are not available (Swedish Institute 1999b).

Although the central government is intricately connected to maintaining health care in Sweden, a number of weaknesses are associated with the system. For example, the following have been identified as systemic weaknesses of the Swedish health care system:

- Lack of integration between primary and hospital care as well as between health and other services.
- Little influence of the consumer.
- Differential outcomes in productivity of hospitals and the services they provide. (Hoffmeyer 1994: 927–928)

The lack of integration among segments of the health care system is a historical problem. As a result, Sweden has a relatively high rate of patient self-referral to hospitals. Patients also have had little say regarding health care. This issue is being addressed: the government has instituted reform efforts that would provide patients with greater physician continuity.

In addition to the problems addressed by Hoffmeyer, Saltman (1998) has identified a number of emerging issues that are of particular relevance to the Swedish health care system. These issues include the following:

- The sustainability of low expenditures
- Potential options for raising new health-sector revenue
- Alternative arrangements to absorb unemployed workers in home and social care jobs

The sustainability of low expenditures refers to the decreasing level of GDP being spent on health care in Sweden. The consequences of reduced spending reflect an increased strain on the system and a shrinking commitment to ensuring equity for all citizens. In particular, Saltman argues that the application of explicit rationing (politically determined) as a result of limited funding will have a greater impact on low-income citizens. Saltman also questions the extent to which middle-class citizens will allow the public system to be fiscally constrained before they respond.

The second issue is of particular concern because it addresses the need of Sweden to raise new revenue for the private sector to compete in an international market. However, any transfer of funds from the public to the private sector will reduce the availability of monies for health care. As Saltman indicates, Sweden has not attempted to transfer a greater percentage of the health care responsibility to individual users through the use of increased co-payments. Rather, Sweden is attempting to create a middle ground response to this issue.

The third issue is the most contentious. Here, Sweden is faced with creating new jobs and reducing the cost of providing for a growing number of unemployed adults. Although these workers could be trained for employment in areas associated with the health care industry, such an outcome is unlikely because most occupations in the health care community are unionized. These workers would thus be opposed as being less skilled and in competition with current workers.

Although systemic reform is natural, Sweden's health care system will retain many of those elements that have defined its basic structure. For example, Saltman (1992) argues that the Swedish health care system will continue to provide universal access to all citizens. In addition, health care will remain a predominantly public responsibility with a single financing source, and primary and preventive services will be expanded (Saltman 1992).

Similar to countries with previous universal access to health care, health outcomes continue to differ among segments of the population. The final section examines these differences on the basis of age, sex, social class, and race and ethnicity.

## THE HEALTH OF THE POPULATION BY AGE, SEX, SOCIAL CLASS, AND RACE AND ETHNICITY

As the previous sections have demonstrated, health care in Sweden represents a structural model considered to be one of the best in the world. Furthermore, Sweden possesses one of the highest life expectancy rates in the world. Nevertheless, the population of Sweden does not share equally in these outcomes. For example, those living in the northern counties experience lower life expectancy rates than residents in the southernmost counties of the country. Historically, Arvidsson and Berglund (1978) demonstrate that mortality rates in Stockholm have been significantly higher when compared with the rest of the country.

This section examines health differences within the Swedish population. As with previous chapters, this section addresses health outcomes relative to four primary sociological variables: age, sex, social class, and race and ethnicity. This section also demonstrates the interrelationship among these variables. Information in this section draws heavily from a report commissioned by the National Board of Health and Welfare (1997).

### Age

The percentage of the Swedish population aged 65 and over is currently the highest in the world. As of 1999, 17.3% of the population was 65 or older (Lassey and Lassey 2001). By 2025, 23.7% of the population is expected to be 65 or older, locating Sweden behind a number of other European nations and Japan (U.S. Bureau of the Census 1992).

The increasing number of elderly in Sweden has not negatively impacted the willingness of the government to ensure their health care needs. Even with system-level reforms of the 1980s and 1990s, the health care needs of the elderly remained a fundamental requirement. In addition to hospital care, older individuals also receive health care from district nurses and home health workers (Swedish Institute 1999b). Home health care in particular has a history in Sweden dating to the 1950s. Although equity in access to home health services is expected, it does not occur in reality. According to Sundstrom and Tortosa (1999), there is a "wide variation in service levels between municipalities" (347). As in other industrialized countries, the elderly consume a disproportionate share of health care costs. For example, Henriksson et al. (1999) report that the elderly in Sweden consume 39% of pharmaceutical sales compared with 6% among those aged 0 to 14, 22% for 15- to 44-year-olds, and 33% for those 45 to 64. Furthermore, the percentage of pharmaceuticals consumed by the elderly is expected to increase as the percentage of the population age 65 and over continues to increase. Given these differences in health care consumption by the elderly, there does not appear to be a generational backlash against the increasingly aged population. Johannesson and Johansson (1996) report that when asked whether older or younger Swedes should be saved, respondents in Sweden were far more likely to support younger Swedes. However, respondent age did not influence the choice, suggesting that beliefs are not generationally bound.

According to the Swedish Institute (1999b), the majority (51%) of elderly live with a spouse, and another 40% live alone. Approximately 8% reside in institutional settings. In 1956, the national government passed the Poor Law, which abolished children's responsibility for their aging adult parents. Thus "the fact that elderly people prefer to receive care from the formal care system than from their own children suggests that the high percentages that have frequent contact with their children are not primarily a consequence of informal care" (Lennartsson 1999: 674).

Furthermore, McCamish-Svensson et al. (1999) found that the availability of formal support systems for the elderly in Sweden does not result in a concomitant reduction in contact and support from family. A cohort analysis of elderly in Goteborg (Svanborg 1988) provides preliminary evidence that the period of time within which social and medical support is needed may be decreasing.

The health of the elderly in Sweden is generally quite good. Not surprisingly, the elderly are more likely to report a chronic illness than their younger counterparts. The elderly are also more likely to report a lower perceived health status (Lennartsson 1999).

It is evident that the health care system of Sweden offers the elderly the opportunity to live their lives in relative comfort and security. As Lassey and Lassey (2001) point out, few in the aging population are subject to living in poverty because social equality among citizens of all ages is greater in Sweden than any other country.

### Sex

As with age, males and females experience differential health opportunities and outcomes in Sweden. For example, life expectancy is greater for females than males, and mortality rates are higher for males than females. Life expectancy differences between females and males are decreasing in Sweden. In 1960, female life expectancy at birth was 74.9 years compared with 71.2 for males. By 1998, life expectancy for females was 81.9 and 76.9 for males (Organization for Economic Cooperation and Development 2000).

According to the National Board of Health and Welfare (1997), the difference between male and female life expectancy is decreasing because of changing lifestyle habits (i.e., smoking). As a result, an increasing number of women are at risk for premature death. However, factors such as biology and living conditions continue to locate greater opportunities for ill health within males compared with females. Furthermore, the National Board of Health and Welfare indicates that although women live longer than men, their social and economic conditions are generally worse than men. For example, the National Board of Health and Welfare (1997) points out that women receive less pay, have less influence in the workplace, and hold more domestic and child-rearing responsibilities. In particular, research by Whitehead, Burstrom, and Diderichsen (2000) suggests that lone mothers experience poorer health outcomes than mothers in two-parent families. Noting that poverty and joblessness are not particularly strong explanations of poorer health, the authors suggest a number of alternatives that include time poverty, poorer quality of work available, and less social support.

In a similar vein, Svensson and Sundh (1999) point out that women are more likely than men to work in the public sector of the Swedish economy. Thus, as a result of recent cutbacks in the public sector, of the 120,000 employees eliminated in county council throughout Sweden, 100,000 were women. Similarly, Manderbacka, Lundberg, and Martikainen (1999) report that women identify their health as slightly poorer than men, and men are more likely to engage in less healthy behaviors. Excess male mortality rates in Sweden have been attributed to a number of factors, including economic growth and labor market factors, medical care, and demographic and consumption factors (Hemstrom 1999a, 1999b).

Although men and women experience differing health outcomes, their utilization rates of prescription drugs is relatively similar. Research by Henriksson et al. (1999) indicates that regardless of age, the distribution of pharmaceutical sales by sex are almost identical. The average cost of prescription drugs, however, differs on the basis of age and sex. Women under the age of 15 had the lowest per capita drug costs, and men over the age of 65 had the highest.

### Social Class

Through various social and economic programs enacted in the latter half of the twentieth century, Sweden has attempted to reduce income differences and, therefore, health outcomes, on the basis of social class. For example, Lahelma et al. (1994) note that as socioeconomic position decreases, the extent of illness increases. The significance of social class is illustrated by the work of Lynch and Greenhouse (1994), who point out that the probability of infant mortality has historically been higher among unskilled workers and farmers and lower among the upper and middle class.

Beginning in the latter 1980s and extending into the early 1990s, Sweden experienced a series of economic problems that resulted in increasing unemployment rates throughout the country. With the slowing of the economy, economic differences between social classes, particularly low- and upper-income earners, has increased. The result has been an increasing differentiation in the health of the population. According to the National Board of Health and Welfare (1997),

More than twice as many male blue-collar workers consider their health is poor as male middle and upper while-collar workers do. Twenty percent more have some long-term illness and more than double this proportion have greatly impaired working ability because of long-term illness. Among female blue-collar workers 60% more than among female white-collar workers at middle and upper levels consider their health as poor, 20% more have a long-term illness and it is just over twice as common that their working ability is impaired. (67)

In addition to health differences between blue- and white-collar workers, growing evidence indicates that unemployment is also related to increased health risk (Brenner and Starrin 1988; Dahlgren and Diderichsen 1986). For example, Catalano, Hansen, and Hartig (1999) report that unemployment among males is correlated with low birth weight.

In addition, unemployment or low income appears to limit one's willingness to access health care if patient charges are required. According to Elofsson, Unden, and Krakau (1998), such charges "can provide a hindrance to seeking care for both financially and psychologically disadvantaged groups and thereby lead to more unequally distributed health care" (1380).

### Race and Ethnicity

Similar to many other European nations, Sweden has been a relatively homogeneous country. Ethnic and racial diversity is a recent phenomenon brought about by the need for an increased workforce. According to Statistics Sweden (1996), the health status of male and female immigrants from Poland, Chile, Iran, and Turkey differed significantly from native Swedes as well as between ethnic groups. For example, the health status of Polish immigrants was most similar to Swedish natives, whereas women from Chile, Iran, and Turkey differed the most from native Swedes. The National Board of Health and Welfare (1997) provides further evidence of health differences between native Swedes and immigrant groups. In a recent report, most immigrant groups experience higher morbidity as well as mortality rates than native Swedes. The report also notes that some immigrant groups (Danish, Norwegian, and Turkish) generally experience better health than their Swedish counterparts.

As the immigrant population in Sweden ages, a new series of issues arise. For example, according to Emami and Ekman (1998), older Iranian immigrants living in Sweden reported feelings of social isolation. As a result, there was "an excessive use of medication and psychosomatic symptoms" (Emami and Ekman 1998: 196). Given these problems, the elderly Iranian immigrants nevertheless considered themselves healthy. More recently, Emami et al. (2000) suggest the need for understanding minority populations' "underlying worldview and patterns of interaction" (184) to more effectively engage them in health promotion efforts.

## CONCLUSION

Universal coverage and utilization of tax revenue for financing locates the Swedish health care system within the Beveridge model. It is a public system with a small, but emerging private sector. The Swedish system represents one of the most comprehensive health care systems in the world. And, until recently, Swedish citizens strongly supported the system. Although public support for the health care system has diminished somewhat, fundamental reform is highly unlikely.

Organizationally, there are three primary levels of government in Sweden: central, county, and local. Although the central government establishes health policy, the 23 county councils and 3 municipal governments are responsible for the administration and provision of health care services. Salaried physicians deliver these services in a regionalized health clinic and hospital system. Recent governmental reforms have attempted to separate providers and purchasers of services in an effort to create a more market-oriented system and patient-friendly system. However, these reform efforts have not had the anticipated effect, in part, because of the cultural framework within which the health care system has been constructed (i.e., the presumption of health equity as a fundamental construct).

Although the Swedish health care system is based on the presumption of health equity, health-related opportunities continue to differ on the basis of age, sex, social class, and race and ethnicity. These differences are manifested in the gross health indicators of life expectancy and infant mortality rates of the country. Nevertheless, the Swedish health care system represents one of the most viable efforts to provide a comprehensive package of health, social, and economic services to its citizens.

## REFERENCES

Abraham, John, and Graham Lewis. 1999. "Harmonising and Competing for Medicines Regulation: How Healthy Are the European Union's System of Drug Approval?" *Social Science & Medicine* 48(11): 1655–1667.

Andersen, Ronald, Bjorn Smedby, and Denny Vagero. 1997. "Sweden: Economy vs. Solidarity." Paper presented at the American Sociological Association Meetings, Toronto, Canada.

Anderson, Gerard F., Jeremy Hurst, Peter Sotir Hussey, and Melissa Jee-Hughes. 2000. "Health Spending and Outcomes: Trends in OECD Countries, 1960–1998." *Health Affairs* 19(3): 150–157.

Anderson, Odin W. 1972. *Health Care: Can There Be Equity: The United States, Sweden, and England.* New York: John Wiley.

Andrain, Charles F. 1998. *Public Health Policies and Social Inequality.* New York: New York University Press.

Angus, Douglas E. 1998. "Health Care Costs: Canada in Perspective." In *Health and Canadian Society: Sociological Perspectives,* 3rd ed., ed. David Coburn, Carl D'Arcy, and George Torrance. Toronto: University of Toronto Press.

Arvidsson, Ola, and Kenneth Berglund. 1978. "Environment and Morbidity." *International Journal of Contemporary Sociology* 15(1–2): 178–193.

Bergman, Sven-Eric. 1998. "Swedish Models of Health Care Reform: A Review and Assessment." *International Journal of Health Planning and Management* 13(2): 91–106.

Bjorkman, James Warner. 1985. "Who Governs the Health Sector? Comparative European and American Experiences with Representation, Participation, and Decentralization." *Comparative Politics* 17: 399–420.

Blendon, Robert J., Robert Leitman, Ian Morrison, and Karen Donelan. 1990. "Satisfaction with Health Systems in Ten Nations." *Health Affairs* 9(2): 185–192.

Borgenhammer, Edgar. 1984. "Health Services in Sweden." In *Comparative Health Systems: Descriptive Analyses of Fourteen National Health Systems,* ed. Marshall W. Raffel. University Park: Pennsylvania State University. Press.

Brenner, Sten-Olof, and Bengt Starrin. 1988. "Unemployment and Health in Sweden: Public Issues and Private Troubles." *Journal of Social Issues* 44(4): 125–140.

Catalano, Ralph, Hans-Tore Hansen, and Terry Hartig. 1999. "The Ecological Effect of Unemployment on the Incidence of Very Low Birthweight in Norway and Sweden." *Journal of Health and Social Behavior* 40(4): 422–428.

Chaulk, C. Patrick. 1994. "Preventive Health Care in Six Countries: Models for Reform?" *Health Care Financing Review* 15(4): 7–19.

Dahlgren, Goran, and Finn Diderichsen. 1986. "Strategies for Equity in Health: Report from Sweden." *International Journal of Health Services* 16(4): 517–537.

Diderichsen, Finn. 1999. "Devolution in Swedish Health Care." *British Medical Journal* 318:1156–1157.

———. 2000. "Sweden." *Journal of Health Politics, Policy and Law.* 25(5): 931–935.

Elofsson, Stig, Anna-Lena Unden, and Ingvar Krakau. 1998. "Patient Charges—A Hindrance to Financially and Psychologically Disadvantaged Groups Seeking Care." *Social Science & Medicine* 46(10): 1375–1380.

Emami, Azita, and Sirkka-Liisa Ekman. 1998. "Living in a Foreign Country in Old Age: Life in Sweden as Experienced by Elderly Iranian Immigrants." *Health Care in Later Life* 3(3): 183–198.

Emami, Azita, et al. 2000. "An Ethnographic Study of a Day Care Center for Iranian Immigrant Seniors." *Western Journal of Nursing Research* 22(2): 169–188.

Federation of County Councils. 1990. *Some Innovative Projects at Swedish County Councils.* Stockholm, Sweden.

Freeman, Richard. 2000. *The Politics of Health in Europe.* Manchester: Manchester University Press.

Freeman, Richard, and Michael Moran. 2000. "Reforming Health Care in Europe." *West European Politics* 23(2): 35–58.

Garpenby, Peter. 1999. Resource Dependency, Doctors and the State: Quality Control in Sweden." *Social Science & Medicine* 49(3): 405–424.

General Accounting Office. 1994. "Prescription Drugs: Spending in Four European Countries." Special Committee on Aging. U.S. Senate. GAO/HEHS-94-30. Washington, DC: Government Printing Office.

Hakansson, Stefan, and Sara Nordling. 1997. "The Health System of Sweden." In *Health Care and Reform in Industrialized Countries,* ed. Marshall W. Raffel. University Park: Pennsylvania State University Press.

Ham, Christopher. 1988. "Governing the Health Sector: Power and Policy Making in the English and Swedish Health Services." *Milbank Quarterly* 66(2): 389–414.

Harrison, Michael I., and Johan Calltrop. 2000. "The Reorientation of Market-Oriented Reforms in Swedish Health-Care:" *Health Policy* 50(3): 219–240.

Hemstrom, Orjan. 1999a. "Explaining Differential Rates of Mortality Decline for Swedish Men and Women: A Time-Series Analysis, 1945–1992." *Social Science & Medicine* 48(12): 1759–1777.

———. 1999b. "Does the Work Environment Contribute to Excess Male Mortality?" *Social Science & Medicine* 49(7): 879–894.

Henriksson, Freddie, Catharina Hjortsberg, and Clas Rehnberg. 1999. "Pharmaceutical Expenditure in Sweden." *Health Policy* 47(2): 125–144.

Hoffmeyer, Ullrich. 1994. "The Health Care System in Sweden." In *Financing Health Care,* Vol. 2, ed. Ullrich K. Hoffmeyer and Thomas R. McCarthy. Dordrecht: Kluwer Academic Publishers.

Immergut, Ellen M. 1992. *Health Politics: Interests and Institutions in Western Europe.* Cambridge: Cambridge University Press.

———. 1999. "Historical and Institutional Foundations of the Swedish Health Care System." In *Health Care Systems in Transition: An International Perspective,* ed. Francis D. Powell and Albert F. Wessen. Thousand Oaks, CA: Sage.

Johannesson, Magnus, and Per-Olov Johansson. 1996. "The Economics of Ageing: On the Attitude of Swedish People to the Distribution of Health Care Resources between the Young and the Old." *Health Policy* 37(4): 153–161.

Lahelma, Eero, Kristiina Manderbacka, Ossi Rahkonen, and Antti Karisto. 1994. Comparisons of Inequalities in Health: Evidence from National Surveys in Finland, Norway, and Sweden." *Social Science & Medicine* 38(4): 517–524.

Lassey, Marie L., William R. Lassey, and Martin J. Jinks. 1997. *Health Care Systems around the World: Characteristics, Issues, Reforms.* Upper Saddle River, NJ: Prentice-Hall.

Lassey, William R., and Marie L. Lassey. 2001. *Quality of Life for Older People: An International Perspective.* Upper Saddle River, NJ: Prentice-Hall.

Lennartsson, Carin. 1999. "Social Ties and Health among the Very Old in Sweden." *Research on Aging* 21(5): 657–681.

Lindbeck, Assar. 1997. "The Swedish Experiment." *Journal of Economic Literature* 35:1273–1319.

Lynch, Katherine, and Joel B. Greenhouse. 1994. "Risk Factors for Infant Mortality in Nineteenth-Century Sweden." *Population Studies* 48(1): 117–133.

Lynch, Matthew J., and Stanley S. Raphael. 1963. *Medicine and the State.* Springfield, IL: Charles C. Thomas.

Manderbacka, Kristiina, Olle Lundberg, and Pekka Martikainen. 1999. "Do Risk Factors and Health Behaviours Contribute to Self-Ratings of Health?" *Social Science & Medicine* 48(12): 1713–1720.

McCamish-Svensson, C., G. Samuelsson, B. Hagberg, T. Svensson, and O. Dehlin. 1999. "Social Relationships and Health as Predictors of Life Satisfaction in Advanced Old Age: Results from a Swedish Longitudinal Study." *International Journal of Aging and Human Development* 48(4): 301–324.

Mossialos, Elias. 1998. "Regulating Expenditures on Medicines in European Union Countries." In *Critical Challenges for Health Care Reform in Europe,* ed. Richard B. Saltman, Josep Figueras, and Constantino Sakellarides. Buckingham, UK: Open University Press.

National Board of Health and Welfare. 1997. *Sweden's Public Health Report: 1997.* Stockholm, Sweden.

Nilsson, Mats. 1997. "Irritation Mounts over Swedish Pharmaceutical Reforms." *The Lancet* 349: 549.

Organization for Economic Cooperation and Development. 1994. *The Reform of Health Care Systems: A Review of Seventeen OECD Countries.* Paris, France.

———. 2000. *OECD Health Data 2000: A Comparative Analysis of 29 Countries.* Paris, France.

Ostman, Lars. 1992. "A Swedish Patient's Experience of the Medical Care System: Ideal and Reality, Power and Dependence." In *Health Care Systems and Their Patients: An International Perspective,* ed. Marilynn M. Rosenthal and Marcel Frenkel. Boulder, CO: Westview Press.

Quaye, Randolph K. 1997. "Struggle for Control: General Practitioners in the Swedish Health Care System." *European Journal of Public Health* 7(3): 248–253.

Rathwell, Tom. 1998. "Implementing Health Care Reform: A Review of Current Experience." In *Critical Challenges for Health Care Reform in Europe,* ed. Richard B. Saltman, Joseph Figueras, and Constantino Sakellarides. Buckingham: Open University Press.

Rehnberg, Clas. 1997. "Sweden." In *Health Care Reform: Learning from International Experience,* ed. Chris Ham. Buckingham: Open University Press.

Riska, Elianne. 1993. "The Medical Profession in the Nordic Countries." In *The Changing Medical Profession: An International Perspective,* ed. Frederic W. Hafferty and John B. McKinlay. New York: Oxford.

Roemer, Milton I. 1991. "The Countries." In *National Health Systems of the World,* Vol. 1. New York: Oxford.

Saltman, Richard B. 1988. "Sweden." In *The International Handbook of Health-Care Systems,* ed. Richard B. Saltman. New York: Greenwood Press.

———. 1990. "Competition and Reform in the Swedish Health System." *Milbank Quarterly* 68(4): 597–618.

———. 1991. "Emerging Trends in the Swedish Health System." *International Journal of Health Services* 21(4): 615–623.

———. 1992. "Recent Health Policy Initiatives in Nordic Countries." *Health Care Financing Review* 13(4): 157–166.

———. 1995. "The Role of Competitive Incentives in Recent Reforms of Northern European Health Systems." In *Health Care Reform through Internal Markets: Experiences and Proposals,* ed. Monique Jerome-Forget, Joseph White, and Joshua M. Wiener. Washington, DC: The Brookings Institution.

———. 1998. "Health Reform in Sweden: The Road Beyond Cost Containment." In *Markets and Health Care: A Comparative Analysis,* ed. Wendy Ranade. London: Longman.

———. 1999. "Evolving Roles of the National and Regional Governments in the Swedish Health Care System." In *Health Care Systems in Transition: An International Experience,* ed. Francis D. Powell and Albert F. Wessen. Thousand Oaks, CA: Sage.

Saltman, Richard B., and Josep Figueras. 1998. "Analyzing the Evidence on European Health Care Reforms." *Health Affairs* 17(2): 85–108.

Somers, Anne R., and Herman M. Somers. 1977. *Health and Health Care: Policies in Perspective.* Germantown, MD: Aspen Systems Corporation.

Statistics Sweden. 1996. "Gaining a Foothold in Sweden: Immigrants from Chile, Iran, Poland and Turkey." Stockholm, Sweden. www.sos.se/fulltext/ 9951–001/9951–001.html. (February 10, 2000).

Sundstrom, Gerdt, and Maria Angeles Tortosa. 1999. "The Effects of Rationing Home-Help Services in Spain and Sweden: A Comparative Analysis." *Ageing and Society* 19: 343–361.

Svanborg, Alvar. 1988. "Cohort Differences in the Goteborg Studies of Swedish 70-Year-Olds." In *Epidemiology and Aging: An International Perspective,* ed. Jacob A. Brody and George L. Maddox. New York: Springer.

Svensson, P.-G. and M. Sundh. 1999. "Public Sector Lay-Offs in Sweden and the Effect on Women's Health." *International Journal of Social Welfare* 8(3): 229–238.

Swedish Institute. 1999a. *The Health Care System in Sweden.* http://www.si.se/ eng/esverige/health. (February 14, 2000).

———. 1999b. *The Care of the Elderly in Sweden.* http://www.sise/eng/ esverige/elderly. (February 14, 2000).

Swedish Medical Association. 2000. *Working in Sweden: Information for Doctors from EU/EEA countries.* National Board of Health and Welfare. Stockholm, Sweden.

U.S. Bureau of the Census. 1992. International Population Reports, P25, 92–3, *An Aging World II.* Washington, DC: Government Printing Office.

von Otto, Casten. 1999. "Cost Control in the Swedish Health Sector." In *Health Care Systems in Transition: An International Perspective,* ed. Francis D. Powell and Albert F. Wessen. Thousand Oaks, CA: Sage.

Wennstrom, Gunnar. 1992. "New Ideological Winds Are Blowing in the Swedish Health Care System." In *Health Care Systems and their Patients: An International Perspective,* ed. Marilynn M. Rosenthal and Marcel Frenkel. Boulder, CO: Westview Press.

Whitehead, Margaret. 1998. "Diffusion of Ideas on Social Inequalities in Health: A European Perspective." *Milbank Quarterly* 76(3): 469–492.

Whitehead, Margaret, Bo Burstrom, and Finn Diderichsen. 2000. "Social Policies and the Pathways to Inequalities in Health: A Comparative Analysis of Lone Mothers in Britain and Sweden." *Social Science & Medicine* 50(2): 255–270.

Wiley, Miriam M. 1994. "Quality of Care and the Reform Agenda in the Acute Hospital Sector." In *Health: Quality and Choice*. Health Policy Studies No. 4. Organization for Economic Cooperation and Development. Paris, France.

World Health Organization. 1996. *Health Care Systems in Transition: Sweden* (preliminary version). Copenhagen, Denmark.

————. 2000. *The World Health Report 2000. Health Systems: Improving Performance.* Geneva, Switzerland.

# CHAPTER 7

# Japan

Japanese health care is delivered, financed, and managed in a sociological environment in which excellence is expected, harmony cultivated, and conflict resolved through negotiation. Japan's government, insurance schemes, hospitals, physicians, and patients seek to carefully maneuver resources, politics, and culture to ensure a balance in the nation's health care system.

(Levin and Wolfson 1989: 312)

## INTRODUCTION

Health care in Japan is provided within a social and political context that ensures stability for all. Universal health care in Japan is a phenomenon that emerged shortly after the end of World War II. Organizationally, the health care system in Japan "is characterized by compulsory universal coverage within a social security framework, financing by employer and individual contributions through non-profit insurance funds, and a combination of public/private ownership of the factors of production" (Angus 1998: 26). Administratively, the system is managed at the regional and local levels of government (Andrain 1998). The Japanese health care system is similar to other industrialized nations in that it represents a work in progress.

Although health care expenditures have increased in Japan, they remain far below the level of the United States. For example, health care expenditures in Japan increased from 3.0% in 1960 to 7.6% in 1998. During the same period of time, health care expenditures as a percentage of GDP increased from 5.1% in 1960 to 13.6% in 1998 in the United States (Organization for Economic Cooperation and Development 2000). Per capita expenditures on health also differed between Japan and the United States. In 1997, the per capita health expenditure in Japan was $1,760 compared with $3,912 in the United States (National Center for Health Statistics 2000). More specifically, Japan spent 28.5% of its total health expenditures on inpatient services in 1997, far below the OECD average of 42.6%. However, physician services consumed 34.4% and prescription drugs 20.8% of total health expenditures. These percentages are higher than the 15.2% and 15.1%, respectively, for OECD countries. Finally, between 1960 and 1998, average annual growth in per capita health care spending in Japan was 6.9% compared with an OECD median of 4.5%. More recently (1990–1998), average growth in per capita health spending increased at an annual rate of 3.5% compared with an OECD median of 2.4% (Anderson et al. 2000).

Nevertheless, although health care costs have remained relatively low by comparison, the Japanese people are not particularly supportive of their health care system. According to Blendon et al. (1990), 29% of Japanese respondents agreed that their health care system needed only minor changes. Forty-seven percent, however, felt the system was in need of fundamental change, and 6% agreed the system should be completely rebuilt. Japan ranked seventh out of the ten industrialized nations in which the findings were gathered. By comparison, only 10% of Americans believed that only minor changes to their health care system were necessary; 60% responded that fundamental changes were necessary; and 29% agreed the health care system needed to be completely rebuilt.

Although relatively recent in its design and implementation, the Japanese system is currently ranked as the tenth best health care system in the world in terms of overall performance (World Health Organization 2000). For example, Japan currently ranks number one in the world for life expectancy rates (see Yanagishita and Guralnik 1988 for an explanation of why Japan surpassed Sweden in life expectancy). In 1998, female life expectancy at birth is 84.0 years, and males have a life expectancy at birth of 77.2 years. At age 65, females can expect to live another 22 years, and males can expect another 17.1 years of life at age 65. The infant mortality rate was 3.6 deaths per 1,000 live births (Organization for Economic Cooperation and Development 2000). Although impressive, Japan is undergoing significant demographic, social, and environmental changes. For example, Japan is not only experiencing a rapidly aging population, but also changes in eating habits and increasing levels of stress. As a result, there is concern regarding the future of its health care system (Yajima and Takayanagi 1998).

## HISTORY OF THE JAPANESE HEALTH CARE SYSTEM

Health care in Japan has evolved over the last fifteen hundred years. The first major effort to influence Japanese medicine occurred in the sixth century C.E. with the introduction of Chinese medicine. A millennium later, Western medicine was introduced. It was not until the latter nineteenth century, however, that Western medicine was integrated into Japanese culture. During the Meiji Restoration (1868–1912), Japan adapted a number of Western initiatives that sped their transition to a modern state (Iglehart 1988). During this period of time, Japan became the first industrialized Eastern nation (Roemer 1991).

The Meiji Restoration period also represented a Westernization of health care in Japan. In 1870, Japan adopted the German health care system. Throughout the ensuing decades, physicians from Japan traveled to Germany for training and German physicians practiced medicine in Japan (Nakahara 1997). An important distinction between the German and Japanese systems is that "Japan does not allow anyone to opt out of the mandated health insurance system to purchase private insurance for benefits covered by the national health insurance program" (Graig 1999: 98).

In 1922, passage of the Health Insurance Law provided the foundation for the current health system. The 1922 law mandated health coverage for miners and factory workers in companies with 15 or more employees. Similar to Germany, dependents were not covered. A revised National Health Insurance Law in 1938 extended coverage to other workers. In 1947, the new Japanese Constitution articulated the role of the state in health care. Article 25 of the Constitution guarantees all citizens "the right to maintain the minimum standards of wholesome and cultured living" (Steslicke 1989: 108). In addition, Article 25 also declares, "In all spheres of life, the state shall use its endeavors for the promotion and extension of social welfare and security, and of public health" (Steslicke 1989: 108). The following year the New Medical Service Law was implemented to regulate health care facilities. By 1958, additional legislation required local governments to provide health care coverage to the unemployed. In 1961, the National Health Insurance Law was implemented. With this legislation, Japan had successfully implemented a universal health care system (Lassey, Lassey, and Jinks 1997). In 1982, the Health and Medical Services for the Aged Law was enacted. Under this law, responsibility for medical spending on the poor was transferred from the national government to employee health insurance plans. A controversial component of the law required the elderly to engage in cost sharing (a co-payment) when receiving health care. The law also attempted to reduce the extraordinary average length of hospital stay associated with Japanese hospitals (Iglehart 1988).

The Japanese health care system continues to undergo reform. Throughout the 1980s and 1990s, reform efforts attempted to contain health care costs. In 1984, a medical services co-payment of 10% was introduced. A year later, Regional Medical Care Plans were introduced. These plans were "to prevent inefficient increases in the number of hospital (beds) and to establish systematic and regular interaction among medical care providers" (Organization for Economic Cooperation and Development 1994: 213).

Other reforms include the 1989 Gold Plan. The purpose of this reform was to improve the health care services provided to a rapidly aging population in Japan. On the one hand, some of the goals of the Gold Plan were to increase the number of workers providing assistance to the elderly (home helpers, day services, and so forth). On the other hand, the Gold Plan had as its goal the inevitable task of bringing the number of elderly bedridden Japanese to zero. The plan also promoted scientific research on aging as well as determining those activities that assist older individuals to lead productive lives (Organization for Economic Cooperation and Development 1994). In essence, the Gold Plan "stressed the need for a nonhospital care delivery system to keep the disabled elderly in the community rather than in institutions" (Usui and Palley 1997: 372). A New Gold Plan was adopted in 1994. This plan, a modification of the 1989 plan, placed greater emphasis on home-help services that would allow the elderly to remain in their community.

More recently, a number of proposals were put forth that would radically alter the health care system of Japan. They include increased co-payments for patients, a separate health plan for the elderly, the use of diagnostic related groups (DRGs), and establishing reference pricing for prescriptions. First, increasing co-payments for patients by allowing physicians to engage in balance billing and hospitals to charge patients directly for certain services have been identified as alternatives to increased taxes. Second, as the number and percentage of the elderly increase, there is a growing sentiment to locate this population in a separate insurance plan funded by taxes and contributions from the elderly themselves. Third, pilot programs have been implemented to determine the utility of diagnostic related groups (DRGs) as a cost control measure for inpatient care. Fourth, reference pricing of prescription drugs is expected to reduce the overall price of medications by eliminating "all profits from drugs for hospitals and physicians" (Ikegami and Campbell 1999: 67).

The Japanese health care system is also unique relative to other industrialized countries in terms of its continued application of *kanpo*, a traditional medical system with origins in China. Essentially, *kanpo* involves the effort to maintain a balance between *yin* and *yang*, represented by *chi*, "a harmonious mixture of these two forces" (Garland 1995: 260). *Kanpo* treatment involves a "regulation of daily habits, of which diet is considered the most important" (Ohnuki-Tierney 1984: 96). The Japanese government has attempted for years to limit the use of *kanpo*, but it has not been successful. Rather, it remains a popular alternative to allopathic medicine, although it is not covered by the health insurance system.

## FINANCING AND DELIVERY OF HEALTH CARE

The Japanese health insurance program is much more complex than the German scheme on which it was modeled. For example, currently some 5,000 independent insurance plans operate in Japan (White 1995). In addition, the financing of the health care system is highly regulated. According to Ikegami (1992a, 1998), the Japanese do not have a choice in insurance funds and cannot opt out of the fund. In addition, the government establishes fee schedules for health services. Planning and administration of the system is through the Minister of Health and Welfare (MOHW).

Health care in Japan is financed through two basic programs: employee health insurance and national health insurance. These two programs can be further subdivided into plans dependent on where one works (much of the following is from Graig 1999; Ikegami 1992a). The financing for each plan also varies. For example, the Employee Health Insurance (EHI) can be subdivided into society-managed plans, government-managed plans, and other (Mutual Aid Associations, Seaman's Insurance, and Day Laborers Insurance). Financing of these plans involves premiums paid by employees and employers ranging from 8.39% of salary to 8.5%. Generally speaking, the premium is split evenly between employers and employees.

The National Health Insurance (NHI) provides health coverage to the self-employed, the unemployed, and employees in small businesses. Financing of the NHI comes from a variety of sources including the local and national government as well as a tax on income. Within the NHI is the Health and Medical Service for the Elderly. This program covers those individuals age 70 and over as well as those age 65 and over if they are bedridden. Recipients in both the EHI and NHI also contribute to the financing of their respective programs through co-payments. These co-payments generally range from 20% to 30% of the cost of inpatient and outpatient services. Health services for the elderly are financed through employment-based plans as well as the government at the local and national levels. According to Nakahara (1997), the national government contributes 20% of the necessary funds to the insurance program for the elderly, with prefectures and local governments each providing 5% of the cost. The bulk of the cost for the elderly program (70%) is borne by health insurance associations. Elderly patients are required to contribute through co-payments for physician visits and hospital inpatient care. According to information provided by the Ministry of Health, Labour and Welfare (2001), the percentage breakdown of persons covered by public insurance scheme is as follows:

30.1%—Government-managed health insurance

26.3%—Association-managed health insurance

8.1%—Mutual Aid Association

35.2%—National Health Insurance

0.3%—Other

Although the income and health of those covered differ by type of plan, benefits are essentially the same for two reasons: "differential subsidies from tax revenues, and a pooling fund for the elderly" (Ikegami and Campbell 1999: 58). For example, the pooling fund for the elderly is achieved through tax revenues at the national and local level as well as from the employment-related insurance funds, which contribute from one-fourth to one-third of their premiums.

Thus, although some differences exist among insurance programs, all citizens are entitled to similar benefits that include "medical and dental care in both inpatient and outpatient settings and expenses related to hospitalization, nursing, and the dispensing of drugs" (Rapp and Shibuya 1994: 603). And, because insurance premiums are based on income rather than health status, the system ensures greater equity (Yoshikawa, Bhattacharya, and Vogt 1996). Nevertheless, "differences in eligibility, administration, cost-sharing, cash benefits and the level of national government subsidy provided" exist (Akaho et al., 1998: 302).

In addition to the social insurance programs, there is a small but growing private insurance sector (Schieber, Poullier, and Greenwald 1992). Supplemental private insurance plans have particularly targeted the hospital needs of the rapidly aging population (Rapp and Shibuya 1994) and those with diseases such as cancer (Campbell and Ikegami 1998).

As noted earlier, the cost of financing the health care system in Japan has been increasing. Although the government has attempted to implement cost-saving measures, health care continues to consume a greater proportion of GDP. Explanations for this increase vary. For example, in addition to an increasingly aged population, Lassey, Lassey, and Jinks (1997) point to increasing rates of chronic diseases such as cancer, the availability of new medical technologies and pharmacological developments, and increased expectations of the public regarding its utilization of health care. However, "the main cause of medical cost increases in recent years has been hospitalization (nursing, room and board, and medical oversights) rather than medications and medical tests" (Hiroi 1996: 69–70).

Regardless of the reason, the Japanese health care system is experiencing a financial strain because a recent recession has meant a greater percentage of GDP is being spent on health care. In conjunction with a stagnating economy, Japan is also experiencing a chronologically older society consuming an increasing proportion of health care expenditures.

Nevertheless, health care costs in Japan are significantly less than the United States. According to Hsiao (1996), Japanese health expenditures are 40% of American expenditures. Hsiao (1996) outlines four reasons why Japanese health care costs are less expensive. First, because of differences in diet and lifestyle, the morbidity rates for most diseases are generally less in Japan than the United States (see also Basch 1990). Second, as a result of differences in health care systems, medical practice styles have resulted "in lower surgical rates, lower hospital admissions, longer average length of stay, and greater use of primary care services" (Hsiao 1996: 48) in Japan when compared with the United States. Expanding on this point, Anders (2000) argues that a point system encouraging higher reimbursement for primary level care and lower reimbursement for the application of high-technology procedures is instrumental in controlling health care costs in Japan. Third, hospital costs are lower in Japan because of fewer personnel per bed as well as lower administrative and drug costs. Fourth, "the health system can be seen as a bazaar where patients can transfer their wealth to physicians, nurses, and technicians in exchange for their labor" (Hsiao 1996: 48).

More specifically, although the average number of staff per bed increased by approximately 50% between 1970 and 1998 in Japan (0.6 to 0.97), the average number of staff per bed doubled during the same time period in the United States (2.27 to 4.55). Thus the United States averages more than four times the number of hospital staff per bed compared with Japan. An example of lifestyle differences between the Japan and the United States is in terms of total caloric and protein intake. In 1988, the total caloric and protein intake in Japan was 3,104 compared with 3,450 in the United States. By 1998, Japanese total caloric and protein intake increased slightly to 3,148 compared with 3,763 for the United States (Organization for Economic Cooperation and Development 2000).

Finally, the Central Social Insurance Medical Care Council, consisting of individuals representing insurers, providers, and the public, makes decisions regarding health care expenditures in Japan. As an advisory body to the Minister of Health, the council establishes fee schedules for all health care providers (physicians and hospitals). In the process, the council considers five basic questions. These questions include how much money providers need and how it will be raised; how much of the increase in health care costs can be covered through savings elsewhere; premium increases; and budget subsidies (Campbell and Ikegami 1998).

## Physicians

The role of the physician in Japan continues to evolve. Although practitioners of traditional Chinese medicine were firmly established by the middle of the eighteenth century, Western medicine was also exerting an influence. Although introduced into Japan in the sixteenth century, it was not until the latter half of the eighteenth century that Western medicine began in earnest. According to Hashimoto (1984), the translation of a German anatomy book by two Japanese scholars in 1774 marked the beginning of Western medicine in Japan. Throughout the nineteenth century, physicians from various Western countries arrived in Japan to teach and assist in the development of medical schools. Nevertheless, in 1849, the central government in Japan limited the study of medicine to traditional Chinese practices (Johansson and Mosk 1987). In 1871, German physicians were invited to teach at the University of Tokyo. Upon completion of their studies, the students were appointed to teaching positions in other institutions throughout Japan. Although the status of some of these institutions was eventually raised to that of university, others, particularly in the private sector, retained their vocational-school status. By 1883, medical licenses were given only to those students who had completed study in Western medicine. In an effort to maintain traditional medical practices, practitioners of Chinese medicine were allowed to continue (Campbell and Ikegami 1998).

The culmination of previous efforts to bring the various factions (Western versus Chinese traditional, private versus hospital based) of physicians together was the establishment of the Japanese Medical Association in 1916. By 1923, membership in the association was compulsory. After World War II, however, the association became voluntary. Although influential, membership in the Japanese Medical Association continues to decline. In 1955, 68% of all physicians were members. By 1992, however, only 52% of physicians maintained membership in the association. Furthermore, private practice physicians are more likely to be members than are hospital-based physicians (Campbell and Ikegami 1998). Given the membership structure, it is not surprising that the association supports the economic interests of private practice physicians by participating in fee schedule negotiations (Ikegami 1994).

Medical education in Japan is similar to Europe. There are currently 80 medical schools throughout the country with the majority controlled by the government (43 by the national government and 8 by local prefectures). Thirty-six percent (29) of the medical schools are private. There is also considerable variation in the quality of the institutions (Levin and Wolfson 1989). The number of students enrolled in medical school declined between 1980 and 1990. In 1980, there were 8,360 students enrolled in medical school (Roemer 1991). By 1990, however, the number had decreased to 7,750. The ratio of physicians to population, however, has improved. In 1980, there were 133 physicians per 100,000 population. By 1988, the number of physicians per 100,000 population had increased to 164 (Tsuda, Aoyama, and Fromm 1994). In 1998, the number of physicians per 100,000 population had again increased to 270. In terms of absolute numbers, there were 96,038 practicing physicians in 1960, 148,815 in 1980, and 238,771 in 1998. The percentage of practicing physicians who are female has also increased. In 1998, 13.9% of practicing physicians were female compared with 9.7% in 1980 and 8.7% in 1960 (Organization for Economic Cooperation and Development 2000). Although the number of physicians continues to increase, Japan, like other industrialized countries, continues to experience a geographical maldistribution of where they practice. According to Nakahara (1997), some areas of the country have over 200 physicians per 100,000 population; other areas have approximately 100 physicians per 100,000 population.

Medical school training in Japan consists of a six-year undergraduate medical education. Upon completion, the physician is licensed to practice medicine. Most physicians spend another two years receiving additional training. Many private practitioners, however, complete another four or five years of medical education in a teaching hospital to earn the doctor of medical science degree. Japan does not certify physicians in specialty areas. Instead, the medical school professor who supervises the training determines the competency of the student in advanced training. Earning the doctor of medical science degree confers additional status but not necessarily a higher income. Rather, physicians who enter private practice generally earn significantly more than hospital-based physicians. Although private practice physicians are all paid a standard fee for services, regardless of their training, they are able to augment their income through the writing and dispensing of prescriptions (Anderson 1998). According to Rodwin and Okamoto (2000), physicians dispense 80% of the drugs in Japan. By the 1990s, pharmaceuticals represented 30% of total health care expenditures (see Suzuki, Ikeda, and Kami 2000 for a defense of the expenditure). As a result of excessive prescribing and dispensing of medications, the Minister of Health and Welfare established a number of policies intended to control the rate of the precribing behavior of physicians. These policies included a reduction in reimbursement levels, incentives for physicians not to dispense medications, and the creation of pharmacies (Rodwin and Okamota 2000).

Although private practitioners generally enjoy higher incomes, they represent a decreasing percentage of the physician population. As a result, the average age of private practitioners is increasing. Perhaps the unique characteristic of private practice physicians in Japan is that they practice out of clinics. These clinics are allowed to have a maximum of 19 beds (20 or more beds is considered a hospital). A single physician and a part- or full-time nurse comprise the staff at these clinics (Levin and Wolfson 1989).

Concomitantly, salaried hospital-based physicians now constitute 55% of the total number of physicians. And, as Greenberg (1996) points out, an increasing number of patients are willing to "wait for over several hours to see a physician in the outpatient department of one of the prestigious teaching hospitals" (95). The willingness of patients to wait illustrates the physician-patient relationship in Japan. Most physicians do not accept appointments. As a result, patients see physicians only when they are sick. The outcome is that patients spend hours waiting to see their physician. The unwillingness of physicians to establish appointment times for patients "reflects the perception and management of time among contemporary Japanese" (Ohnuki-Tierney 1984: 176). Once in an examination room, however, the visit only lasts approximately five minutes (Campbell 1996). A further defining characteristic of the physician-patient relationship is that patients rarely seek a second opinion because it represents "a questioning of his/her competence" (Akiyama 1992: 172). However, a negative characteristic of the physician-patient relationship has been an increase in Japan medical malpractice litigation (Nakajima et al. 2001). For example, in 1970 there were 0.09 suits per 100 physicians. In 1998, there were 0.25 suits per 100 physicians. Nevertheless, these numbers remain far below litigation rates in the United States.

Finally, although the number of physicians graduating from medical school doubled from 4,000 to 8,000 between 1980 and 1990, rural areas remain underrepresented. In addition, Eisenberg and Foster (1996) suggest changes regarding how physicians are trained. For example, Japan needs more general practitioners who can focus on primary and preventive care. They also suggest an increase in the number of residency programs and board certification of those physicians who are trained as specialists.

### Hospitals

Historically, Western-style hospitals in Japan date to 1557. Because of a self-imposed isolation from Western influence, however, the advent of a significant Western influence was not felt until the mid-1800s. Japan has also accorded more prestige to public, rather than private hospitals (Nakahara 1997).

Hospitals in Japan can be classified into one of five categories: general, tuberculosis, mental, communicable diseases, and leprosy. As of 1992 there were 8,877 general hospitals, 11 tuberculosis, 1,052 mental hospitals, 7 for communicable diseases, and 16 leprosy facilities. A further classification by sponsorship reveals that hospitals exist at all governmental levels (national, prefectural, and municipal). In addition, public service corporations, health insurance associations, private medical service associations, and individuals sponsor hospitals. Physicians who staff hospitals are employed full time and are on salary.

There is an abundance of hospital beds in Japan. According to the Organization for Economic Cooperation and Development (2000), the number of inpatient care beds per 1,000 population increased from 9.0 in 1960 to 16.5 per 1,000 population in 1998. By comparison, the United States had 9.2 inpatient beds per 1,000 population in 1960 and 3.7 in 1998. The average length of stay in Japanese hospitals is also much longer than other industrialized countries. The average length of stay of 40.8 days in Japan is more than three times greater than Germany, at 12.0 days. Japan has a greater average length of hospital stay for a number of reasons, which include social and cultural factors as well as administrative decision making. Muramatsu and Liang (1996) suggest that, compared with the United States, the longer average length of stay in Japan is the result of physician decision making and patient and family requests, as well as differences in availability of hospital personnel. That is, Japan generally has fewer full-time personnel than American hospitals. A recent assessment of staffing levels found that over 40% of hospitals were below national requirements. More importantly, 3% of the hospitals were staffed at less than half of what was required by law (Wocher 2000). In addition to staffing, hospitals are also experiencing problems of institutional efficiency. For example, the average length of hospital stay creates a shortage of available beds. Attempting to increase capacity, Kawabuchi (2000) argues that if Japan utilized diagnostic related groups (DRGs), the result would be increased bed capacity and a limit on hospital costs. These outcomes are considered increasingly important given the rapidly growing number of elderly within the country. Patient satisfaction with hospital care also appears to depend on what they expected as a result of their care (an emphasis on technology or interpersonal care). Regardless of their expectations, patient satisfaction was related to "doctor's clinical competence, and recovery from distress and anxiety" (Tokunaga, Imanaka, and Nobutomo 2000: 398).

## CURRENT REALITIES AND ROLE OF THE STATE

Because of political, economic, and demographic changes, the Japanese health care system continues to experience structural modifications. At the present time, the Japanese health care system is beginning to experience perhaps its greatest challenge: providing for the rapidly increasing number of aging citizens. Although this problem is addressed in greater detail in the following section, it is important to note the impact of chronological age on the health care system. In addition to greater utilization of the health care system, the elderly are increasingly reliant on the system for support once provided through the family. At the same time, the younger population has increased their expectation of the health care system. As a result, there is concern regarding the ability of the health care system to contain costs (Ikegami 1994). Ikegami (1992b) points to three problems with the health care system, including limits to the fee scheduling approach, rigidity of the system, and quality.

The Japanese government has identified a number of areas in need of immediate reform. According to Ikegami and Campbell (1999), they include the following:

- Increasing patients' share of costs
- Creating an independent insurance plan for the elderly
- Introducing inclusive payments for acute inpatient care
- Setting reference prices for drugs

These government proposals have not received support from the Japanese population. Ikegami and Campbell (1999) outline a number of reasons for their likely demise. First, efforts to increase patient co-payments appear unlikely because most of the medical claims are the result of a small minority of the population. Second, it is not feasible financially to assume the aging population could bear the cost of covering the cost of insurance. Furthermore, other insurance carriers would still be responsible to cover some of the cost of providing health care to the elderly. In addition, local governments would be considered responsible for insuring the elderly and possibly incurring any deficits as a result. Implementation of diagnostic related groups would also be difficult, because most hospitals do not have data sufficient to assess such plans. Also, current payment methods are based on staffing ratios, thus impacting those facilities with large nursing staffs. Finally, implementation of reference pricing is not expected because current drug pricing has already had some impact regarding the cost of prescription drugs.

Although Ikegami and Campbell (1999) do not expect other reform efforts to succeed in contemporary Japan, they identify two areas within the current health care system that they believe are desperately in need of reform. First is the inequality of burden. Although the health care system is relatively egalitarian, there are considerable differences in premiums that reflect the health of the insurers. Because of structural changes within the Japanese economy, premium differences could widen as less healthy insurers are forced to increase premiums at a faster rate than healthy insurers. The second area of immediate reform is the quality of care. This problem exists on a number of levels within the health care community. For example, external evaluations of physicians are generally nonexistent, as are specialty boards that would establish standards of knowledge. Structurally, Japanese health care is biased toward physicians in an office practice. As a result, many hospitals are not sufficiently reimbursed for the services they perform, resulting in overcrowding and understaffing (see also Ikegami 1992a).

Within all of these problems is the issue of whether or not the government of Japan can continue financing the current system of health care. As the older age population increases, health care expenditures will rise, thus increasing the cost of health care on the government (Faruqee and Muhleisen 2001). Perhaps more than anything else, the demographic shift occurring in Japan defines a future reality for all industrialized nations.

## THE HEALTH OF THE POPULATION BY AGE, SEX, SOCIAL CLASS, AND RACE AND ETHNICITY

Although health care in Japan represents an effort to ensure equality, differences in access and outcomes exist. This section addresses these differences and their consequences, in particular the impact of a rapidly aging population and governmental efforts to control health care costs without jeopardizing the health of the elderly or others within the population. For example, between 1973 and 1992, the government provided free medical care to those aged 70 and over. However, the government was forced to abandon the effort because of cost (Hoshino 1996).

### Age

As noted earlier, Japan has the longest life expectancy of any industrialized nation. Shortly, Japan will become the "oldest" country in the world with the largest percentage of its population age 65 and over. In addition, the location of this aging population is not uniform throughout the country. Currently, rural areas of Japan have relatively high concentrations of the aging population. The growth in the older age population throughout the first two decades of the twenty-first century will be in the industrialized urban centers of Japan (Nishio 1994).

According to the U.S. Bureau of the Census (1992), the percentage of the population age 65 and over in Japan is expected to increase from 11.8% in 1990 to 21.3% in 2010 and 26.7% in 2025. Putting this in perspective, it took 24 years (1970–1994) for the over-age 65 population to double in Japan (7–14%). By comparison, it took the United States 75 years to double its aging population from 7% to 14% (Usui and Palley 1997). Perhaps even more dramatic is the percentage increase among those age 80 and over. In 1990, 2.4% of the population was over the age of 80. By 2025, this is projected to increase to 9.3% of the population. By comparison, 4.3% of the American population is expected to be over the age of 80 by 2025. This demographic shift will have long-range implications for the health care system of Japan. For example, in 1998, there were 17 people age 80 and over for every 100 in the 50 to 64 age category. By 2025, this ratio is expected to increase to 42 (Velkoff and Lawson 1998).

Japan has attempted to alleviate health access and cost problems associated with an aging population. Within the past two decades the government has adopted various reforms. For example, in 1982, the Elderly Health Care System was implemented. The purpose of this program was to provide a centralized financial pool from which health care costs for the elderly would be paid. The intent of the program was to address the inequalities of age associated with the thousands of insurers throughout Japan (Okamoto 1996). In 1989, implementation of the Gold Plan was intended to enhance services for the elderly (particularly in-home services) in Japan. The plan emerged as the result of changes occurring within the family structure and assumed familial responsibilities (Adachi, Lubben, and Tsukada 1996). The goals of the Gold Plan include the following:

(1) urgent development of in-home services for the aged in municipalities,

(2) reduction of bedridden aged people to zero,

(3) establishment of a Longevity Social Welfare Fund to enhance the welfare of the aged,

(4) urgent development of institutional facilities for the aged,

(5) promotion of measures to enhance productive aging,

(6) promotion of gerontological research, and

(7) development of comprehensive welfare institutions for the aged. (Adachi, Lubben, and Tsukada 1996: 149)

Because of rapid growth in participants and cost, Japan continues to modify health-related programs for the elderly. In early 2000, Japan instituted a new program, Long-Term Care Insurance (LTCI). The program is financed through mandatory contributions from all workers age 40 and over. All older individuals (age 65 and over) and all those aged 40 to 64 with a disability are eligible. Essentially, the program shifts responsibility for services from the family to the government with administration of the program at the municipal level. Movement away from family support is the result of a number of factors including a change in values about caring for the elderly and the increasing role of women in paid employment (Ogawa and Retherford 1997). Services under LTCI are categorized into institutional care and community-based care. Institutional care consists of nursing homes, health facilities for the elderly, and specific long-term care beds in hospitals. Community-based care includes home help services that include such activity as housekeeping and bathing (Campbell and Ikegami 1998, 2000).

　　Given these historical efforts, publicly financed long-term care services in Japan have proved difficult because of systemic deficiencies (e.g., staffing levels) (see, for example, Ikegami and Yamada 1996; Imai 1998; Lassey and Lassey 2001). Recent economic problems in Japan have prompted researchers to examine the willingness of Japanese workers and the elderly to pay for long-term care insurance (see, for example, Kitajima 1999). In addition, the rapidly aging population is creating intergenerational tension as the cost of providing health care to the elderly impacts the economic survival of the country. In fact, one company "refused to pay more than half of its share of insurance premiums, arguing that the system was unfair on a company that had so many young employees" (Watts 2000: 2075).

## Sex

Although research is not as extensive, health outcomes also differ between males and females in Japan. For instance, as in other industrialized countries, women in Japan experience longer life expectancy than men. Examining life expectancy differences between males and females over time in Japan, Bass (1996) illustrates the growing differentiation between males and females. In 1947, life expectancy was 4.8 years greater for females. By 1993, however, women were living almost 6.5 years longer than men. One consequence of greater life expectancy among women in Japan as elsewhere is the greater likelihood of institutionalization in later life. Whereas males between the ages of 60 to 74 are slightly more likely than females to be institutionalized in Japan, females aged 75 and over are significantly more likely than males to be institutionalized (Velkoff and Lawson 1998). Also, Riley (1990) reports that females experienced a greater increase than males in morbidity rates between 1955 and 1985 in almost all age categories. During the same time period, however, females experienced a generally greater decline in mortality rates than men. Middle-aged Japanese women are also less likely to utilize health care services than women in other age categories and middle-aged women in other cultures. According to Lock (1996), "more than 60% of the women in the present study have never discussed menopause...with a doctor, and only 17% have brought what they characterize as symptoms...to the attention of a physician" (212).

## Social Class

Social class is not widely applied in Japan. Hashimoto (2000), however, argues that the class structure of Japan "has become increasingly close to pure capitalism, with the old middle class declining and the new middle class and working class increasing" (61). Nevertheless, access to health care in Japan is relatively equal, regardless of income, occupation, employment status, and so forth (Andrain 1998). Although the economic burden associated with access to health care is not the same for all, differences are generally minor. For example, Campbell (1996) argues that out-of-pocket expenses between a 10% and 30% co-payment for a physician visit is about $5. As a result, there is considerable equity in access and burden, regardless of health or economic status. According to Campbell

(1996), "the healthy and wealthy subsidize the poor and the sick" (259). Nevertheless, Mosk and Johansson (1986) demonstrate that a declining mortality rate is related to increased income. Cockerham, Hattori, and Yamori (2000), however, question the relationship between income and health in Japan. They argue that the greatest life expectancy in Japan is on Okinawa, the prefecture with the lowest per capita income. The reason cited for the increased life expectancy on Okinawa is lifestyle and the social context within which it is performed.

### Race and Ethnicity

Race and ethnicity is a particularly difficult area to address because Japan is ethnically homogeneous. In addition, Japan has a limited immigrant population (Lassey, Lassey, and Jinks 1997). According to Henshall (1999), currently some 1.5 million legal immigrants live in Japan and an unknown number of illegal immigrants. Koreans represent the largest foreign group followed by Chinese and Brazilians. Although discrimination against foreigners is illegal, informal discriminatory practices persist. Job opportunities for foreigners are also limited. For example, employment for legal Koreans is usually "in the entertainment or service industries, or small-scale manufacturing" with illegal Koreans in "casual laboring" (Henshall 1999: 64). Thus, in addition to subtle forms of discrimination within Japanese society, foreigners may experience health care problems because of their occupation and consequent participation in the corresponding health insurance scheme.

### CONCLUSION

The Japanese health care system shares characteristics of the German social insurance model, although the Japanese system remains unique. For instance, unlike the German model, Japanese cannot opt out and enter the private market. In addition, the Japanese system represents a unique effort to ensure equity of access and burden among all participants. Begun in 1961, the system continues to provide quality health care at one of the lowest per capita rates in the industrialized world. The quality of the health care system is demonstrated by the greatest life expectancy for males and females in the world.

The Japanese health care system is financed through a number of insurance plans. The basic insurance plans include Employee Health Insurance (EHI), National Health Insurance (NHI), and health service for the elderly. Employee plans are further subdivided into plans operated by large corporations, the government-managed program that covers employees in small and medium-sized companies, the Seaman's Insurance, and Mutual Aid Associations. The National Health Insurance program provides coverage for the self-employed, farmers, the unemployed, retirees, and their dependents. Local government authorities administer the National Health Insurance program. Although premiums differ among insurance plans, health care coverage is essentially the same for all Japanese, regardless of characteristics such as age, sex, or social class position. A small private health care sector provides supplementary insurance, particularly for the elderly and those with specific diseases.

The delivery of services continues to evolve in Japan. Although the number of physicians continues to increase, efforts to reduce the number of specialists and locate a greater number of physicians in primary care areas is an ongoing challenge. Physicians in Japan are categorized as either in private practice or are hospital based. Physicians in private practice supplement their relatively low incomes by prescribing medications to their patients. These physicians also operate clinics (with up to 19 beds). The number of physicians in private practice is decreasing. The number of salaried hospital-based physicians, however, is increasing.

One of the unique features of the Japanese health care system is the number of hospital beds available and the average length of stay. Although other industrialized countries have reduced the number of available hospital beds, Japan has been increasing its supply. Because of cultural, familial, and administrative factors, the average length of stay in Japan is significantly longer than any other industrialized country.

The relatively low cost of health care in Japan and the rapidly aging population have created a number of immediate problems for the system. Various reform efforts, including increasing co-payments, have been implemented to curb the growing cost of care. Nevertheless, the Japanese health care system is characterized as providing equality of access and burden in addition to a relatively low cost of care.

## REFERENCES

Adachi, Kiyoshi, James E. Lubben, and Noriko Tsukada. 1996. "Expansion of Formalized In-Home Services for Japan's Aged." *Journal of Aging & Social Policy* 8(2–3): 147–159.

Akaho, Eiichi, G. D. Coffin, and T. Kusano. 1998. "A Proposed Optimal Health Care System Based on a Comparative Study Conducted between Canada and Japan." *Canadian Journal of Public Health* 89(5): 301–307.

Akiyama, Hiroko, 1992. "Twenty Years of Care in Japan: Sakuji Uehara, as Told to Hiroko Akiyama by Toshiomi Asahi." In *Health Care Systems and Their Patients: An International Perspective*, ed. Marilynn M. Rosenthal and Marcel Frenkel. Boulder, CO: Westview Press.

Anders, Robert L. 2000. "Japan's Healthcare System." *Journal of Nursing Administration* 30(4): 169–172.

Anderson, Gerard F. 1998. *Multinational Comparisons of Health Care: Expenditures, Coverage, and Outcomes.* New York: Commonwealth Fund.

Anderson, Gerard F., Jeremy Hurst, Peter Sotir Hussey, and Melissa Jee-Hughes. 2000. "Health Spending and Outcomes: Trends in OECD Countries, 1960–1998." *Health Affairs* 19(3): 150–157.

Andrain, Charles F. 1998. *Public Health Policies and Social Inequality.* New York: New York University Press.

Angus, Douglas E. 1998. "Health Care Costs: Canada in Perspective." In *Health and Canadian Society: Sociological Perspectives,* 3rd ed., ed. David Coburn, Carl D'Arcy, and George Torrance. Toronto: University of Toronto Press.

Basch, Paul F. 1990. *Textbook of International Health.* New York: Oxford.

Bass, Scott A. 1996. "Introduction: Japan's Aging Society." In *Public Policy and the Old Age Revolution in Japan,* ed. Scott A. Bass, Robert Morris, and Masato Oka. New York: Haworth Press.

Blendon, Robert J., Robert Leitman, Ian Morrison, and Karen Donelan. 1990. "Satisfaction with Health Systems in Ten Nations." *Health Affairs* 9(2): 185–192.

Campbell, John Creighton. 1996. "The Egalitarian Health Insurance System." In *Containing Health Care Costs in Japan,* ed. Naoki Ikegami and John Creighton Campbell. Ann Arbor: University of Michigan Press.

Campbell, John Creighton, and Naoki Ikegami. 1998. *The Art of Balance in Health Policy: Maintaining Japan's Low-Cost, Egalitarian System.* Cambridge: Cambridge University Press.

Campbell, Ruth. 1996. "The Three Minute Cure: Doctors and Elderly Patients in Japan." In *Containing Health Care Costs in Japan,* ed. Naoki Ikegami and John Creighton Campbell. Ann Arbor: University of Michigan Press.

Cockerham, William C., Hiroyuki Hattori, and Yukio Yamori. 2000. "The Social Gradient in Life Expectancy: The Contrary Case of Okinawa in Japan." *Social Science & Medicine* 51(1): 115–122.

Eisenberg, John M., and Nancy Foster. 1996. "Afterword: Quality and Cost in Japanese and U.S. Medical Care." In *Containing Health Care Costs in Japan,* ed. Naoki Ikegami and John Creighton Campbell. Ann Arbor: University of Michigan Press.

Faruqee, Hamid, and Martin Muhleisen. 2001. "Japan: Demographic Shock and Fiscal Sustainability." International Monetary Fund Working Paper. WP/01/40.

Garland, T. Neal. 1995. "Major Orientations in Japanese Health Care." In *Global Perspectives on Health Care,* ed. Eugene B. Gallagher and Janardan Subedi. Englewood Cliffs, NJ: Prentice-Hall.

Graig, Laurene A. 1999. *Health of Nations: An International Perspective on U.S. Health Care Reform,* 3rd ed. Washington, DC: Congressional Quarterly.

Greenberg, George D. 1996. "Afterword: Costs—The Micro Perspective." In *Containing Health Care Costs in Japan,* ed. Naoki Ikegami and John Creighton Campbell. Ann Arbor: University of Michigan Press.

Hashimoto, Kenji. 2000. "Class Structure in Contemporary Japan." *International Journal of Sociology* 30(1): 37–64.

Hashimoto, Masami. 1984. "Health Services in Japan." In *Comparative Health Systems: Descriptive Analyses of Fourteen National Health Systems,* ed. Marshall W. Raffel. University Park: Pennsylvania State University Press.

Henshall, Kenneth. 1999. *Dimensions of Japanese Society: Gender, Margins and Mainstream.* New York: St. Martin's.

Hiroi, Yoshinori. 1996. "The 'Natural Increase' and Cost Control." In *Containing Health Care Costs in Japan*, ed. Naoki Ikegami and John Creighton Campbell. Ann Arbor: University of Michigan Press.

Hoshino, Shinya. 1996. "Paying for Health and Social Care of the Elderly." *Journal of Aging & Social Policy* 8(2–3): 37–55.

Hsiao, William C. 1996. "Afterword: Costs—The Macro Perspective." In *Containing Health Care Costs in Japan*, ed. Naoki Ikegami and John Creighton Campbell. Ann Arbor: University of Michigan Press.

Iglehart, John K. 1988. "Japan's Medical Care System." *New England Journal of Medicine* 319: 807–812.

Ikegami, Naoki. 1992a. Japan: Maintaining Equity through Regulated Fees." *Journal of Health Politics, Policy and Law* 17(4): 689–713.

———. 1992b. "The Economics of Health Care in Japan." *Science* 258: 614–618.

———. 1994. "Efficiency and Effectiveness in Health Care." *Daedalus* 123(4): 113–125.

———. 1998. "Overview: Health Care in Japan." In *Containing Health Care Costs in Japan*, ed. Naoki Ikegami and John Creighton Campbell. Ann Arbor: University of Michigan Press.

Ikegami, Naoki, and John Creighton Campbell. 1999. "Health Care Reform in Japan: The Virtues of Muddling Through." *Health Affairs* 18(3): 56–75.

Ikegami, Naoki, and Takeshi Yamada. 1996. "Comparison of Long-Term Care for the Elderly between Japan and the United States." In *Containing Health Care Costs in Japan*, ed. Kaoki Ikegami and John Creighton Campbell. Ann Arbor: University of Michigan Press.

Imai, Kaori. 1998. "Bed-Ridden Elderly in Japan: Social Progress and Care for the Elderly." *International Journal of Aging and Human Development* 46(2): 157–170.

Johansson, S. Ryan, and Carl Mosk. 1987. "Exposure, Resistance and Life Expectancy: Disease and Death during the Economic Development of Japan, 1900–1960." *Population Studies* 41(2): 207–235.

Kawabuchi, Koicki. 2000. "Patient Systems and Considerations of Case Mix—Are Diagnosis-Related Groups Applicable in Japan?" *PharmaEconomics* 18 (Suppl. 1): 95–110.

Kitajima, Tsutomu. 1999. "Willingness to Pay for Long-Term Care Insurance System in a Municipality in Tokyo." *Asia-Pacific Journal of Public Health* 11(2): 101–108.

Lassey, William R., and Marie L. Lassey. 2001. *Quality of Life for Older People: An International Perspective*. Upper Saddle River, NJ: Prentice-Hall.

Lassey, Marie L., William R. Lassey, and Martin J. Jinks. 1997. *Health Care Systems around the World: Characteristics, Issues, Reforms*. Upper Saddle River, NJ: Prentice-Hall.

Levin, Peter J., and Jay Wolfson. 1989. "Health Care in the Balance: Japanese Eurythmy." *Hospital and Health Services Administration* 34(3): 311–323.

Lock, Margaret. 1996. "Keeping Pressure Off the Japanese Health Care System: The Contribution of Middle-Aged Women." In *Containing Health Care Costs in Japan*, ed. Naoki Ikegami and John Creighton Campbell. Ann Arbor: University of Michigan Press.

Ministry of Health, Labour and Welfare. (2001). "Health Insurance. General Characteristics." National Institute of Population and Social Security Research. www.jpss.go.jp/english. (April 8, 2001).

Mosk, Carl, and S. Ryan Johansson. 1986. "Income and Mortality: Evidence from Modern Japan." *Population and Development Review* 12(3): 415–440.

Muramatsu, Naoko, and Jersey Liang. 1996. "Comparison of Hospital Length of Stay and Charges between Japan and the United States." In *Containing Health Care Costs in Japan*, ed. Naoki Ikegami and John Creighton Campbell. Ann Arbor: University of Michigan Press.

Nakahara, Toshitaka. 1997. "The Health System of Japan." In *Health Care and Reform in Industrialized Countries*, ed. Marshall W. Raffel. University Park: Pennsylvania State University Press.

Nakajima, Kazue, et al. 2001. "Medical Malpractice and Legal Resolution Systems in Japan." *Journal of the American Medical Association* 285(12): 1632–1640.

National Center for Health Statistics. 2000. *Health United States, 2000*. Washington, DC: Government Printing Office.

Nishio, Harry Kaneharu. 1994. "Japan's Welfare Vision: Dealing with a Rapidly Increasing Elderly Population." In *The Graying of the World: Who Will Care for the Frail Elderly?* ed. Laura Katz Olson. Binghamton, NY: Haworth Press.

Ogawa, Naohiro, and Robert D. Retherford. 1997. "Shifting Costs of Caring for the Elderly Back to Families in Japan: Will It Work?" *Population and Development Review* 23(1): 59–94.

Ohnuki-Tierney, Emiko. 1984. *Illness and Culture in Contemporary Japan: An Anthropological View*. Cambridge: Cambridge University Press.

Okamoto, AtoZ. 1996. "Japan's Financing System for Health Care of the Elderly." *Journal of Aging & Social Policy* 8(2–3): 25–35.

Organization for Economic Cooperation and Development. 1994. *The Reform of Health Care Systems: A Review of Seventeen OECD Countries*. Paris, France.

———. 2000. *OECD Health Data 2000: A Comparative Analysis of 29 Countries*. Paris, France.

Rapp, Richard T., and Kyoko Shibuya. 1994. "The Health Care System in Japan." In *Financing Health Care*, Vol. 1, ed. Ullrich K. Hoffmeyer and Thomas R. McCarthy. Dodrecht, Netherlands: Kluwer Academic Publishers.

Riley, James C. 1990. "The Risk of Being Sick: Morbidity Trends in Four Countries." *Population and Development Review* 16(3): 403–432.

Rodwin, Marc A., and Etsuji Okamoto. 2000. "In Japan and the United States: Lessons for the United States." *Journal of Health Politics, Policy and Law* 25(2): 343–375.

Roemer, Milton I. 1991. *The Countries*. Vol. 1 of *National Health Systems of the World*. New York: Oxford University Press.

Schieber, George J., Jean-Pierre Poullier, and Leslie M. Greenwald. 1992. "U.S. Health Expenditure Performance: An International Comparison and Data Update." *Health Care Financing Review* 13(4): 1–87.

Steslicke, William E. 1989. "Health Care and the Japanese State." In *Success and Crisis in National Health Systems: A Comparative Approach*, ed. Mark G. Field. New York: Routledge.

Suzuki, Ritsuro, Masayuki Ikeda, and Masahiro Kami. 2000. "Japanese Physicians and Public Respect." *The Lancet* 356: 598.

Tokunaga, Junya, Yuichi Imanaka, and Noichi Nobutomo. 2000. "Effects of Patient Demands on Satisfaction with Japanese Hospital Care." *International Journal for Quality in Health Care* 12(5): 395–401.

Tsuda, Toshihide, Hideyasu Aoyama, and Jack Fromm. 1994. "Primary Health Care in Japan and the United States." *Social Science & Medicine* 38(4): 489–495.

U.S. Bureau of the Census. 1992. International Population Reports, P25, 92–3, *An Aging World II*. Washington, DC: Government Printing Office.

Usui, Chikako, and Howard A. Palley. 1997. "The Development of Social Policy for the Elderly in Japan." *Social Service Review* 71(3): 360–381.

Velkoff, Victoria A., and Valeria A. Lawson. 1998. "Gender and Aging: Caregiving." International Brief. IB/98–3. U.S. Department of Commerce. Economics and Statistics Administration. Bureau of the Census. Washington, DC: Government Printing Office.

Watts, Jonathan. 2000. "Japan Makes Older People Contribute towards Their Health Care." *The Lancet* 356: 2075.

White, Joseph. 1995. *Competing Solutions: American Health Care Proposals and International Experience*. Washington, DC: The Brookings Institution.

Wocher, John C. 2000. "Healthcare Reform and Medical Errors in Japan—Are We Walking Backwards?" *Journal of the Japan Hospital Association* 19:11–14.

World Health Organization. 2000. *The World Health Report 2000: Health Systems: Improving Performance*. Geneva, Switzerland.

Yajima, Ricko, and Nazue Takayanagi. 1998. "The Japanese Health Care System: Citizen Complaints, Citizen Possibilities." *Journal of Health and Human Service Administration* 20(4): 502–519.

Yanagishita, Machiko, and Jack M. Guralnik. 1988. "Changing Mortality Patterns That Led Life Expectancy in Japan to Surpass Sweden's: 1972–1982." *Demography* 25(4): 611–624.

Yoshikawa, Aki, Jayanta Bhattacharya, and William B. Vogt. 1996. *Health Economics of Japan: Patients, Doctors, and Hospitals under a Universal Health Insurance System*. Tokyo: University of Tokyo Press.

# CHAPTER 8

# Conclusion

> The expression "health system" is but a shorthand word, a convention, to delineate or to differentiate or to identify the totality of formal efforts, commitments, personnel, institutions, economic resources, research efforts (both basic and applied) that a nation-state or a society earmarks or devotes to illness, premature mortality, incapacitation, prevention, rehabilitation, and other health-related problems.
>
> (Field 1989: 10)

## INTRODUCTION

In chapter 1, I argued that health care systems worldwide are experiencing some of the most difficult challenges in their history. These challenges threaten to disrupt the social and economic relationships on which modern health care is established. Attempting to compare these challenges among health care systems and the nations that employ them is at best difficult for a number of reasons. For example, international comparisons are problematic because

- Data are generally not comparable.
- Systems' performance cannot be easily evaluated because of our inability to measure health outcomes.
- It is difficult to measure and control for social, medical, cultural, demographic, and economic differences across countries.
- Transferability of policies across countries is difficult. (Schieber and Poullier 1990: 9)

However, Roemer (1991) underscores the importance of examining differences among health care systems when he suggests that knowing how others function assists in understanding one's own system. More specifically, knowing what works in one system may provide the impetus for others to emulate. In other words, a comparative analysis of health care systems provides evidence that goals such as health equality are attainable across systems. Thus, relative to international comparisons, "one might pose specific questions to different systems, such as, how they handle aging and dying, or what the relationship is between coercion to compliance and health outcomes in societies ascribing to different social ethics" (Unschuld 1979: 527).

Employing such an approach, I have identified three challenges applicable to the six countries and three health care systems addressed in this book. One challenge is represented by outcomes associated with the historical development of the society (i.e., a shift in the demographic structure toward an aging population). If the availability of medical technologies is generally similar throughout the industrialized world (White 1995), then a second challenge is represented by outcomes associated with the technological advancement of a society (i.e., the extent to which medical technologies are utilized). Finally, a third challenge is represented by outcomes associated with the growing social and economic inequality characteristic of industrialized nations. Combined, these challenges represent a formidable task for any health care system. The interconnection of these challenges also underscores another problem for all health care systems: the cost.

## THE IMPACT OF AGING POPULATIONS ON HEALTH CARE SYSTEMS

The populations of the industrialized world are aging. However, location in this demographic shift varies by country. Table 8.1 identifies past and projected percentages of the age 65 and over population for the six countries discussed in this book. Table 8.2 presents past and projected percentages of the age 80 and over populations for the same countries.

The data in these tables reveal that the United States will remain a relatively young society in comparison with other industrialized nations. Nevertheless, the United States appears more concerned with this population shift than other industrialized nations as it attempts to micromanage access to health care among the elderly. American elderly, in comparison with Canada and the United Kingdom, report more difficulty paying medical bills, affording prescription drugs, becoming a burden on their family, and being concerned about the cost of long-term care (Schoen et al. 2000). Demographically, the percentage of the population age 65 and over in Canada and the United Kingdom is equal to or

**Table 8.1**
**Percentage of the Population Age 65 and Over, Select Countries, 1970–2025**

| Country | 1970 | 1990 | 2010 | 2025 |
|---|---|---|---|---|
| United States | 9.8% | 12.5% | 13.4% | 18.7% |
| Canada | 7.9% | 11.5% | 14.3% | 20.7% |
| Great Britain | 12.9% | 15.7% | 17.1% | 21.5% |
| Germany | 13.2% | 15.0% | 20.4% | 24.4% |
| Sweden | 13.7% | 18.0% | 19.6% | 23.7% |
| Japan | 7.1% | 11.8% | 21.3% | 26.7% |

*Source:* U.S. Bureau of the Census. 1992. International Population Reports, P25, 92-3, *An Aging World II.* Table 1. Washington, DC: Government Printing Office.

**Table 8.2**
**Percentage of the Population Age 80 and Over, Select Countries, 1970–2025**

| Country | 1970 | 1990 | 2010 | 2025 |
|---|---|---|---|---|
| United States | 1.8% | 2.8% | 3.8% | 4.3% |
| Canada | 1.5% | 2.4% | 4.1% | 5.2% |
| Great Britain | 2.2% | 3.7% | 5.1% | 6.3% |
| Germany | 1.9% | 3.8% | 5.2% | 7.7% |
| Sweden | 2.3% | 4.4% | 5.9% | 7.5% |
| Japan | 0.9% | 2.4% | 5.7% | 9.3% |

*Source:* U.S. Bureau of the Census, International Population Reports, P25, 92-3, *An Aging World II.* Table 1. Washington, DC: Government Printing Office.

greater than the United States. Furthermore, these countries spend significantly less than the United States on health care. Germany and Japan, the two countries representative of the Bismarck model of health care, are projected to have the largest percentage of their population age 65 and over. They are also projected to have a larger percentage of their population in the age 80 and over category than other nations presented in this book.

As the populations of all industrialized countries continue to age, it is expected that they will exert increasing pressure on the health care system through greater utilization rates leading to higher costs. An examination of OECD countries by Narine (2000), however, did not find a significant relationship between age and rising health expenditures.

Examining five of the six countries in this book, Anderson and Hussey (1999) point out that there is no correlation "between the percentage of GDP spent on health care for people age 65 and older and the percentage of the population in this age group" (3). In addition, all of these countries experience greater life expectancy and lower infant mortality rates when compared with the United States.

In conclusion, the impact of population aging on health care systems (particularly cost) appears to be minimal (Anderson and Hussey 1999). It is also apparent that relative to the entrepreneurial model, the Bismarck and Beveridge models of health care systems provide a more efficient level of care to their aging populations. Although the public-oriented Bismarck and Beveridge models have initiated various reforms in an effort to control the health care costs of their aging populations, they remain grounded in the belief structure on which their systems were founded.

## THE IMPACT OF MEDICAL TECHNOLOGY ON HEALTH CARE SYSTEMS

As demonstrated throughout previous chapters, the six countries presented in this book have adopted varying levels of medical technology within their health care systems. The following illustrates system-level differences regarding the application of medical technology within the general population in the mid- to late 1990s. Although the entrepreneurial American health care system spends considerably more per capita and as a percentage of GDP on health care, it ranks second, relative to the other five countries in this book, in the number of MRIs per million population, fourth in the number of CT scanners, and sixth in the total expenditure on pharmaceuticals and other durable goods as a percentage of total expenditure on health. Countries (Japan and Germany) within the Bismarck health system model ranked first and fourth, respectively, in the number of MRI units per million population, and first and second, respectively, in the number of CT scanners per million population. They also rank first and fifth, respectively, in terms of total expenditure on pharmaceuticals and other nondurables as a percentage of total expenditure on health. Countries with a Beveridge health system model (Canada, Great Britain, and Sweden) ranked sixth, fifth, and third, respectively, in the number of MRI units per million population, and fifth, sixth, and third, respectively, in the number of CT scanners per million population. They also ranked third, second, and fourth, respectively, in terms of total expenditure on pharmaceuticals and other nondurables as a percentage of total expenditure on health (Organization for Economic Cooperation and Development 2000).

Clearly, countries in the Bismarck model generally have a significant level of medical technologies available. Concomitantly, countries with a Beveridge model of health care generally have fewer medical technologies available per million population. Countries utilizing the Beveridge model generally spend a lower percentage of GDP on health care than countries in the Bismarck or entrepreneurial models. As a result, countries employing the Beveridge model of health care systems need to develop a balance between their levels of health care spending and availability of medical technologies.

## THE IMPACT OF ECONOMIC INEQUALITY ON
## HEALTH CARE SYSTEMS

All health care systems are negatively impacted by economic inequality. Although most industrialized nations provide their citizens with health care, regardless of ability to pay, differences in access and health-related outcomes persist, thus creating the third major challenge to health care systems.

Measuring the impact of economic inequality on health care systems is difficult. One problem is the lack of sufficient data addressing the relationship between social class position and health care (Krieger and Fee 1994), particularly in the United States. However, if criteria such as the number of uninsured citizens within each country are examined, significant differences are apparent. In the entrepreneurial American health care system, 15.8% of all Americans or 17.9% of Americans under the age of 65 were uninsured. Disaggregating these numbers by age, almost one-third (32%) of 19- to 24-year-olds did not have health insurance in the first half of 1999. In addition, 25% of 25- to 29-year-olds were uninsured, as were 23% of 18-year-olds. These percentages declined to 19% for 30- to 34-year-olds, 16% for 35- to 64-year-olds, and 14% for children under 18. By race and ethnic background, 14% of whites were uninsured as were 21% of blacks and 36% of Hispanics. Stated differently, 12.6% of the population is Hispanic, and they constitute 25.2% of the uninsured. Blacks are also overrepresented among the uninsured. Black Americans represent 13.1% of the population but 15.2% of the uninsured. Finally, 69.6% of the population is white, and they make up 54.6% of the uninsured (Medical Expenditure Panel Survey 2001).

By comparison, all of the other industrialized countries in this book provide universal health care coverage to all citizens through either tax-funded or insurance-based systems (Saltman and Figueras 1998). In Germany, however, less than 1% of the population is voluntarily uninsured. The European countries examined in this book are also actively involved in addressing inequalities. According to Whitehead (1998), "the European Union (EU)...has identified research on inequalities in health as a priority for its public health program" (472). On a more general level, Pfaff (1990) argues that services in industrialized nations with a Beveridge or Bismarck model of health care system "are more equitably distributed in relation to health" (22). Again, by comparison, the entrepreneurial American system has done little to address economic inequalities and their impact on health care. For example, one of the few national studies linking health status and socioeconomic status indicates that as income decreases, the greater is the identification of health status as fair or poor (National Center for Health Statistics 2000).

The preceding discussion illustrates system-level differences regarding the prioritization of these challenges as well as efforts to ameliorate their

**Figure 8.1**
**Prioritization of Demographic, Technological, and Economic Inequality Challenges on Health Care Systems, by Country**

| Country | Demography | Technology | Inequality |
|---|---|---|---|
| United States | 1 | 2 | 3 |
| Canada | 3 | 2 | 1 |
| Great Britain | 3 | 2 | 1 |
| Germany | 2 | 3 | 1 |
| Sweden | 3 | 2 | 1 |
| Japan | 2 | 3 | 1 |

effects. Figure 8.1 illustrates my rank ordering of the three challenges by the six countries examined in this book.

Relative to the health care systems presented throughout this book, the entrepreneurial American system has identified the demographic challenge of an aging population as the most important challenge and classified the outcomes of social and economic inequality as the least important (see, for example, Light 2000a). Interestingly, the other five countries have, for some time, considered the outcomes of social and economic inequality as the most important challenge facing their respective health care systems (for example, see Whitehead 1998 regarding Great Britain and Sweden). In addition, I would argue that the Bismarck (social insurance) model of Germany and Japan considers outcomes associated with their respective demographic challenges second and challenges associated with technology outcomes third. In contrast, the Beveridge (health service) model of Canada, Great Britain, and Sweden are more likely to identify challenges associated with technology outcomes as the second most important challenge and demography third.

The purpose of these rankings is twofold. First, the rankings locate the position of each country relative to the others. Perhaps more important is the location of the health care systems each country has adopted relative to the others. Although each country has created its unique adaptation to its health care system, aggregated health outcomes reflect distinct differences among health care systems.

These rankings reflect not only differences among system models, but also the ideological and political frameworks from which the models have emerged. For example, Navarro (1993) argues that "in order to understand the medical care sector one needs to understand the political, social, and economic macro forces that shape and condition the funding, organization, governance, efficiency, and effectiveness of the health services" (5). Thus health care in the United States is informally structured and pluralistic. In Great Britain, health care is centralized, whereas it has been decentralized to the regional and local authorities in Sweden (Bjorkman 1985; see also Hollingsworth, Hage, and Hanneman 1990). The role of the state is particularly noted in a World Health Organization (1997) analysis of European health care systems. According to the report, a number of European nations are reforming their health care systems in an effort to improve access to services.

Relative to all three challenges is the issue of health care cost. Although health care costs differ among countries, the U.S. expenditure is greater than any other country in the industrialized world. In 1998, the United States spent 13.6% of GDP on health care. By comparison, countries within the Beveridge model spent, on average, 8.2% of GDP on health care, whereas countries within the Bismarck model averaged 9.1%. More specifically, Canada, Sweden, and Great Britain spent 9.5%, 8.4%, and 6.7%, respectively, and Germany and Japan spent 10.6% and 7.6%, respectively (U.S. Bureau of the Census 2000). However, as the previous data has indicated, the entrepreneurial American system has poorer outcome data than the Beveridge or Bismarck models. The United States also has a smaller percentage of older age citizens than the other industrialized nations. And the number of advanced medical technologies such as MRI and CT scanners per million population locates the United States in roughly the middle of the countries examined here. Thus the demographic shift and medical technology does not represent a greater challenge for the United States when compared with other industrialized nations.

Examining how well health care system models perform offers another assessment of their response to the three challenges identified earlier. According to the World Health Organization (2000), whatever the health care model, the system should attempt to achieve the following goals: "good health, responsiveness to the expectations of the population, and fairness of financial contribution" (xi). Furthermore, the WHO argues that attainment of these goals depends on four functions: service provision, resource generation, financing, and stewardship. How well a health care system performs these functions influences the extent to which they will meet the goals. An overall ranking of health care systems throughout the world by the World Health Organization illustrates the extent to which these goals are being met.

The ranking of member countries of the Organization for Economic Cooperation and Development by type of health care system reveals outcome differences by model. All of the countries in the Bismarck model were within the top 25 systems in the world with an average system performance score of 14.9. Also, all but one health care system in the Beveridge model were in the top 35. Countries in this model had an average system performance score of 21.1. The two countries in the entrepreneurial model (the United States and Turkey) were ranked 37th and 70th, respectively, for an average system performance score of 53.5. Thus the differences and similarities that exist among these three health care system models and the countries within which they are embodied leads to a fundamental question regarding the future of health care systems: where are they headed?

## CONVERGENCE/DIVERGENCE OF HEALTH CARE SYSTEMS

As stated earlier, the three primary models of health care currently employed throughout the industrialized world reflect ideological and political differences that exist among nations (see, for example, Ertler et al. 1987 for an analysis of indicators associated with the social context of health care systems). These models also reflect an evolutionary process that is the culmination of reform efforts throughout the twentieth century. The World Health Organization (2000) identifies three generations of system-level reform. The first generation was "the founding of national health care systems, and the extension to middle income nations of social insurance systems, mostly in the 1940s and 1950s" (13). The second generation of system reform addressed the application of primary health care through public health measures. Whereas the first two generations of system reform were supply oriented, the third generation is demand oriented. These reforms are characterized by efforts such as allowing "money [to] follow the patient" (World Health Organization 2000: 15). In a similar vein, Gallagher (1989) identifies a number of propositions associated with the evolution of health care systems.

Although the current health care systems reflect different social, political, and economic realities, they represent an increasing attempt at the cross-fertilization of knowledge (see, for example, chapters 12 and 13 in Matcha 2001). For instance, Whiteford and Nixon (2000) argue that health system reform is an outcome of increasing globalization. Whatever the reason, many of the countries with either a Beveridge or Bismarck model are experimenting with internal markets (Jerome-Forget, White, and Wiener 1995). Other examples include attempts by many European nations to improve the efficiency of their health care systems through greater competition and regionalization (Freeman 2000; Freeman and Moran 2000; van de Ven 1996). These reform efforts reflect "the *extent* to which market forces should replace a state system of control" (Scheil-Adlung 1998: 104). One result of these efforts is a shifting of health care costs to consumers and a greater increase in inequality (Light 2000a). At the same time, the entrepreneurial American system has incrementally increased the level of public financing through recent state-run programs such as Child Health Plus. Some states are also studying how best to implement statewide universal health care. The American Congress has also begun debate regarding how best to reduce the impact of prescription drug costs for the elderly. Nevertheless, the United States remains the only industrialized nation in which citizens do not have universal access to health care. The entrepreneurial American system is also the most expensive and the most ineffective (based on the 43 million Americans without health insurance).

The evolution of health care systems worldwide has prompted debate regarding their eventual outcome. The primary focus of this debate is whether health care systems are converging into a homogeneous framework or maintaining their distinctive characteristics. For instance, Mechanic and Rochefort (1996) identify six areas of convergence. They include cost control and improved efficiency, health promotion and health behavior, health inequalities, growth of technology and primary care, greater involvement of patients, and, finally, addressing the impact and needs of an aging population (see also Lassey, Lassey, and Jinks 1997).

Although these factors "put common burdens on systems throughout the world" (Mechanic and Rochefort 1996: 266), their eventual outcomes are, nonetheless, still the result of the political, economic, and social belief structures that regulate the health care system. For example, Jacobs (1998) contends that although the United Kingdom, Sweden, and the Netherlands incorporated the same policy instrument, their policy content is dissimilar, as a result of differing policy goals.

Similarly, Luft (1994) also argues that efforts to integrate an HMO model into systems other than the United States should first "inquire as to what is the perceived local problem...[and then] consider the HMO not as a 'package' to be imported, but as a set of lessons concerning the use of incentives to shape medical care delivery" (59). On the issue of HMOs, however, Abel-Smith (1988) instead asks why HMOs in the United States have not been able to provide the level of population coverage that HMOs attained throughout Europe in the early to mid-twentieth century.

His answers address a number of basic differences between the United States and European health care. For example, early HMOs in Europe were generally not private commercial ventures. At the same time, physician organizations were not well developed and HMO patients had not established relationships with physicians. Thus, although a recent Organization for Economic Cooperation and Development (1994) report argued that system-level reform efforts are converging, the report also states "there appears to be no relationship between success in containing costs and ways of organizing services" (Organization for Economic Cooperation and Development 1994: 49). In addition, Raffel (1997) argues that the creation of cross-national solutions for health care systems does not imply homogenization of systems. For example, research by Mackenbach (1991) did not find a relationship between a country's level of health expenditure and system effectiveness (mortality reduction).

Given the system-level changes occurring throughout all health care models, the question of whether they are converging is probably the wrong question. Although there is a greater willingness to experiment with reform efforts, differences among health care systems will not disappear (Andrain 1998; Graig 1999). Saltman and Figueras (1998) present what is perhaps the most concise statement against convergence. They point out that "suggestions of convergence among the health care systems of developed countries—beyond the transference of narrowly technical mechanisms—appears to be misplaced" (105). Similarly, after an extensive analysis in which he located a number of health care systems on a market-minimized/market-maximized continuum, Anderson (1989) concluded, "a single model does not seem to be practical" (162), and Ludvigsen and Roberts (1996) state that relative to the European community, "no attempt is likely to be made in the foreseeable future to harmonize health care or to try to put in place a European health service" (81). As a result, the future of health care systems appears to be one of realignment rather than convergence. According to Hirsch (1982), effective health care systems should exhibit six characteristics that include the following:

- Equal access
- Response to demographic and morbidity trends
- ·Flexibility to address the uncertainty associated with technologies and other cultural trends
- The most effective application of available resources
- The ability to address those problems interrelated with health such as poverty, housing, and adequate nutrition
- Ongoing self-evaluation and flexibility to change when needed

These characteristics address the need for continued system reorientation rather than convergence toward homogeneity. Similarly, these characteristics provide a framework for the emergence of developing health care systems in the former Soviet Union and Eastern bloc nations.

## IMPLICATIONS FOR THE DEVELOPING WORLD, RUSSIA, AND THE FORMER EASTERN BLOC COUNTRIES OF EUROPE

With the collapse of the former Soviet Union and Eastern bloc nations in the late 1980s and early 1990s, efforts have been ongoing to redesign their health care systems. The state model, as created in the former Soviet Union, was built on the premise of guaranteed universal health access from birth to death financed through the state (Field 1995). Although state-run health care systems can be effective (Cereseto and Waitzkin 1986; Elling 1980, 1989), they have not remained a vital component within the ever-changing landscape of Eastern Europe and the former Soviet Union. As Field (1990) points out, "the *principle* of socialized medicine is one of the most popular and accepted aspects of the Soviet system. It is its execution that is faulted" (144). The Cuban system, however, remains as an example of an effective state-run health care system (Matcha 2000). In fact, the World Bank recently extolled the Cuban health care system as an example for other developing nations.

Throughout Eastern Europe and the former Soviet Union, state-run health care systems are being transformed primarily into a mixture of American entrepreneurial and Bismarck social insurance schemes. Whether such arrangements are in the best health interests of the affected populations remains uncertain. What we know is that the state model, particularly in the former Soviet Union, was not adequately funded throughout much of its 70-year existence. During the 1960s, it has been estimated that approximately 6% of GDP was spent on health care. By the early 1990s, that had declined to around 2% to 3%. Available demographic indexes from the mid-1960s to the 1980s indicate a decreasing life expectancy and increased infant mortality rate (Mezentseva and Rjmachevskaya 1990). These trends have continued and become increasingly problematic with the passage of time. Providing an in-depth analysis of health in Russia and the former Eastern bloc nations, Cockerham (1999) examines the reasons for their declining health status. By the 1990s, the population of Russia began to decline as the number of deaths outpaced births. Nevertheless, these outcomes were not solely the result of a flawed health care system. Rather, the health problems of Russia are also the result of "a 'life style' or way or quality of life, a deteriorating environment, and a sense of despair about an increasingly meaningless world" (Field 1995: 1476).

With the adoption of the Russian Health Insurance Act (HIA) in 1991, health care was transferred from the state as a universal government service to private insurance (McKeehan 1995). Composed of 28 articles, the HIA decentralized health care into a network of health agencies. Health insurance was required of all workers and financed with payments to insurance funds. By 1993, however, the act was refined. In essence, the HIA was a combination of the Clinton Health Security Act and the Canadian system.

The 1993 Health Insurance Act followed the Canadian model of guaranteeing universal access through public health insurance. In keeping an employer payroll tax as the primary financing mechanism rather than direct taxation, the 1993 HIA followed the American model. (McKeehan 1995: 191)

Implementation of these reforms, however, remains problematic given the economic conditions experienced by most Russian citizens. With high levels of unemployment, poverty, and the associated social stresses, the health care system of Russia will experience considerable strain, making reform efforts even more difficult. As Lassey, Lassey, and Jinks (1997) report, collecting funds from employers remains difficult because one-seventh are either bankrupt or experiencing financial difficulty.

In addition to changes within the state model in Russia, health care reform efforts are also occurring within the former Eastern European countries. Poland, for example, continues to discuss the evolution of its state-run health care system into a mix of public and private interests. Similar to the Health Insurance Act in Russia, Poland has discussed the creation of a social insurance health care system. According to Roemer (1994), health system financing would consist of employment-based insurance funds as well as government funding of insurance premiums for those unable to pay (unemployed, disabled, and so forth). However, as of 1992, Poland had not enacted health system legislation. Although other sectors of the economy have been privatized, the population of Poland has not pushed for similar changes in the health care system. Unlike the Russian system, the percentage of GDP spent on health care in Poland gradually increased throughout the 1990s. In 1990, 5.3% of GDP was spent on health care. By 1998, it had increased to 6.4% of GDP (Organization for Economic Cooperation and Development 2000). However, economic problems throughout the 1990s diminished the standard of living and, consequently, the health status of the population (Wnuk-Lipinski 1990).

By contrast, Hungary initiated a number of reforms following the downfall of the Communist Party in 1989. The newly elected parliament enacted a number of basic principles outlining the role of government in the health care system. Although health care is a right, the new government places greater emphasis on individual responsibility, shifting costs toward a social insurance program (Angelus 1992). More specifically, health system changes focused on improving the status of family physicians as well as how they are paid for their services. The method of payment has changed from salary to capitation. Funding for the new health care system and pensions is expected to come from employers and employees. However, the current economic problems encountered in Hungary and other former Eastern bloc countries have made this transition difficult (Roemer 1994). As a result, the percentage of GDP spent on health care decreased from 7.3 in 1991 to 6.8 in 1998 (Organization for Economic Cooperation and Development 2000). Overall health status also declined in Hungary throughout the decade of the 1990s (Orosz 1990).

As the former Soviet Union and Eastern bloc nations continue to experience economic transitions, their former state-run health care systems will also be transformed. What is apparent, however, is that the emerging health care systems represent an amalgam of the three basic models already in existence. Although these new systems reflect the malleability of health system application, they also reflect the narrow range of options available.

## THE NEED FOR NEW MODELS OF HEALTH CARE SYSTEMS

As previous sections in this chapter illustrate, health care systems of the industrialized nations remain structured around three basic models: entrepreneurial, social insurance (Bismarck), and the tax-supported Beveridge. Although variations of the latter two have incorporated some of the market strategies of the entrepreneurial model, these modifications have not substantially altered their basic structure. Although a multiplicity of explanations can be advanced to explain the lack of intersystem integration, it is important to realize that the specific features of a health care system are not necessarily transferable. In other words, what may work in one country may not be applicable in another (Wessen 1999). Furthermore, the Bismarck and Beveridge models remain committed to their basic system-level principles of equity and fairness (see, for example, Whitehead 1992). At the same time, however, these principles have come under attack by conservative critics who wish to Americanize their health care systems, thereby creating a multitiered and increasingly expensive system.

The most frustrating reforms are those that have not occurred. For example, adaptations of the equity and fairness principles at the heart of the European models continue to remain elusive within the entrepreneurial model. Analyzing national political support for a universal health care system in the United States, Matcha and Sessing-Matcha (2001) report that 30 out of the 835 Democratic and Republican congressional candidates identified support for universal health care on their Web sites. Among the 30 candidates, most (23) were Democratic challengers, with 6 Democratic incumbents and 1 independent. Most of the challengers (20) lost the election, and all incumbents were reelected. In addition, 2 Democratic senators up for reelection in the 2002 and 2004 election cycle also identified support for universal health care on their Web sites. The 107th Congress thus has 8 members of the House of Representatives (out of 435) and 4 senators (out of 100) who identified their support for universal health care (in other words, 2.2% of Congress). Although other members of Congress may support an alternative to the current entrepreneurial system, they did not mention it as an issue on their campaign Web sites. Given these statistics, it is difficult to imagine the issues of fairness and equity as understood within the context of universal health care as a major political issue in the United States for the foreseeable future.

Given the overall lack of system-level integration between the entrepreneurial and European models, it is apparent that health system convergence has not had widespread appeal on either side of the Atlantic. Research suggests that the contribution of a market-based American system for countries such as Great Britain and Sweden may in fact be quite negative. Increased levels of competition in England and Sweden "may have lain the foundations for an explosion of health care costs" (Glennerster and Matsaganis 1994: 249–250). Indeed, both countries have recently reduced their reliance on market reforms (Saltman and Figueras 1997).

Nevertheless, escalating health care costs will eventually force the United States and other industrialized nations to address the immediate and long-term impact of a number of issues relevant to their health care systems. For example, reform efforts can generally be dichotomized into either continued government support for equity and fairness or increasing differentiation of health care access through market reforms (see, for example, Davis 1998).

Given the problems associated with all health care systems, current models and their various configurations are not adequate to address the sociodemographic and sociopolitical changes occurring in the United States and other industrialized nations. Thus it is imperative to begin developing alternative health care systems that reflect the current realities of many developed nations. The construction of a new series of health care systems, however, remains problematic for a number of reasons. For example, Hsiao (1992) argues that creating an optimal structure for health care systems is difficult because of three obstacles: "(1) health care systems are a means to an end, (2) the ideological debate between those who favor free enterprise and those who believe in the merits of government planning, and (3) inadequate knowledge and insufficient empirical information" (614).

Given the lack of system convergence and system-level problems when reforms are attempted, alternative system models should be country specific. However, regardless of the health care system, the creation of alternative, or at least variations, on current systems requires acknowledgment of two basic realities. First, access to health care without concomitant access to other life-affirming opportunities (education, jobs, housing, and so forth) will not produce a healthy and productive society—in other words, an issue of fairness. A second basic reality is that the increasing cost of health care to the individual and society is a by-product of a profit-oriented service delivery system (particularly medical technologies). These realities can be distilled to represent two basic societal outcomes associated with health care systems: inequality and profit or equality and nonprofit. How societies address these two realities will define their options within the current health care system as well as alternatives outside the current system.

Although the European models emphasize fairness, they also allow varying degrees of service delivery profit. In contrast, the American entrepreneurial system allows extensive service delivery profit at the expense of fairness (i.e., universal access to health care and other life-affirming opportunities). The American entrepreneurial system and variants of the European model have mistakenly attempted to control escalating costs by increased price competition and altering patient behavior. The problem is that "price competition in health care is so fraught with dangers of selective marketing, inequalities, worsening care, and ironically higher costs, it is unclear how many countries will employ it and for how long" (Light 2000b: 394). Rather, these models would be better served by controlling the profit incentive associated with health services, particularly medical technologies such as pharmaceuticals (Bell 1989).

Radical alteration of current health care systems in the industrialized world does not appear imminent. Rather, efforts will continue to pursue incremental changes to alleviate the growing pressure for more direct action. Eventually, however, the industrialized world will be forced to make decisions regarding how and to whom health care services will be distributed. At the same time, these countries will also be forced to reconsider the role of economic profit from the creation and delivery of these services. Whether these decisions are based on political expediency, rational economics, or the social good remains to be seen.

## CONCLUSION

This chapter assessed the three basic health care systems discussed throughout this book: entrepreneurial, Bismarck (social insurance), and Beveridge. Building on earlier evaluations of system-level differences, the chapter examined in depth the impact of population aging, medical technology, and economic inequality on the three health care systems. Identifying outcomes associated with these challenges, I offered a ranking of the three systems relative to these universal challenges. Briefly, I argued that the entrepreneurial system identifies outcomes associated with demographics as the most important, and outcomes associated with issues of economic and social equality as the least important. Countries within the Bismarck and Beveridge models all consider issues associated with equality the most important challenge. The least important challenge among countries with the social insurance (Bismarck) system are outcomes associated with medical technologies, whereas countries with the Beveridge system consider outcomes associated with demographics the least important. I argued that these outcomes reflect the ideological and political frameworks of the countries involved.

This chapter also addressed the question of health system convergence and/or divergence. Given the cross-fertilization of knowledge regarding health care, system-level convergence would appear a likely outcome. Although proponents of convergence offer evidence supporting their contention, others suggest the issue is that of system adaptation. For purposes of comparison, I also discussed the impact of changes from state-run health care systems to modified social insurance models in the former Soviet Union and in the former Eastern European nations of Poland and Hungary.

Finally, this chapter examined the need for new models of health care systems. Analyzing the overall lack of system integration, it was apparent that although efforts have been made to Americanize various aspects of the European health care models, there is limited support for implementing specific features from one system to another. Although it is believed the development of country-specific alternative models would provide greater enhancement of health opportunities, the context within which issues such as system fairness and profitability are determined remains a crucial, but unknown element.

## REFERENCES

Abel-Smith, Brian. 1988. "The Rise and Decline of the Early HMOs: Some International Experiences." *Milbank Quarterly* 66(4): 694–719.

Anderson, Gerard F., and Peter S. Hussey. 1999. "Health and Population Aging: A Multinational Comparison." New York: Commonwealth Fund.

Anderson, Odin. 1989. *The Health Services Continuum in Democratic States: An Inquiry into Solvable Problems.* Ann Arbor, MI: Health Administration Press.

Andrain, Charles F. 1998. *Public Health Policies and Social Inequality.* New York: Washington Square Press.

Angelus, Tamas. 1992. "Consensus and Health Policy in Hungary." *Journal of Medicine and Philosophy* 17: 455–462.

Bell, Susan E. 1989. "Technology in Medicine: Development, Diffusion, and Health Policy." In *Handbook of Medical Sociology,* 4th ed., ed. Howard E. Freeman and Sol Levine. Englewood Cliffs, NJ: Prentice-Hall.

Bjorkman, James Warner. 1985. "Who Governs the Health Sector?" *Comparative Politics* 17: 399–420.

Cereseto, S., and H. Waitzkin. 1986. "Capitalism, Socialism, and the Physical Quality of Life." *International Journal of Health Services* 16: 643–658.

Cockerham, William C. 1999. *Health and Social Change in Russia and Eastern Europe.* New York: Routledge.

Davis, Karen. 1998. "Common Concerns: International Issues in Health Care System Reform." President's Message. 1998 Annual Report. New York: Commonwealth Fund.

Elling, Ray. 1980. *Cross-National Study of Health Systems.* New Brunswick, NJ: Transaction.

———. 1989. "The Comparison of Health Systems in World-System Perspective." *Research in the Sociology of Health Care* 8: 207–226.

Ertler, Wolfgang, H. Schmidt, J. M. Treyth, and H. Wintersberger. 1987. "The Social Dimensions of Health and Health Care: An International Comparison." *Research in the Sociology of Health Care* 5: 1–62.

Field, Mark G. 1989. "Introduction." In *Success and Crisis in National Health Systems: A Comparative Approach,* ed. Mark G. Field. New York: Routledge.

———. 1990. "Noble Purpose, Grand Design, Flawed Execution, Mixed Results: Soviet Socialized Medicine after Seventy Years." *American Journal of Public Health* 80(2): 144–145.

———. 1995. "The Health Crisis in the Former Soviet Union: A Report From the 'Post-War' Zone." *Social Science & Medicine* 41(11): 1469–1478.

Freeman, Richard. 2000. *The Politics of Health in Europe.* Manchester, UK: Manchester University Press.

Freeman, Richard, and Michael Moran. 2000. "Reforming Health Care in Europe." In Special Issue on Recasting European Welfare States, ed. Maurizio Ferrera and Martin Rhodes. *West European Politics* 23(2): 35–58.

Gallagher, Eugene B. 1989. "A Two-Pronged Foray into the Comparative Study of Health Care Systems." *Sociological Focus* 22(3): 173–180.

Glennerster, Howard, and Manos Matsaganis. 1994. "The English and Swedish Health Care Reforms." *International Journal of Health Services* 24(2): 231–251.

Graig, Laurene A. 1999. *Health of Nations: An International Perspective on U.S. Health Care Reform,* 3rd ed. Washington, DC: Congressional Quarterly.

Hirsch, Gary B. 1982. "A Systems View of Health Services and Their Reorientation: Summary of the Conference Proceedings and Background Papers." In *Reorienting Health Systems: Application of a Systems Approach,* ed. Charles O. Pannenborg, Albert van der Werff, Gary B. Hirsch, and Keith Barnard. New York: Plenum Press.

Hollingsworth, J. Rogers, Jerald Hage, and Robert A. Hanneman. 1990. *State Intervention in Medical Care: Consequences for Britain, France, Sweden, and the United States, 1890–1970.* Ithaca, NY: Cornell University Press.

Hsiao, William C. 1992. "Comparing Health Care Systems: What Nations Can Learn from One Another." *Journal of Health Politics, Policy and Law* 17(4): 613–636.

Jacobs, Alan. 1998. "Seeing Difference: Market Health Reform in Europe." *Journal of Health Politics, Policy and Law* 23(1): 1–33.

Jerome-Forget, Monique, Joseph White, and Joshua M. Wiener. 1995. *Health Care Reform through Internal Markets: Experience and Proposals.* Montreal, Quebec: The Institute for Research on Public Policy.

Krieger, N., and E. Fee. 1994. "Social Class: The Missing Link in U.S. Health Data." *International Journal of Health Services* 24(1): 25–44.

Lassey, Marie L., William R. Lassey, and Martin J. Jinks. 1997. *Health Care Systems around the World: Characteristics, Issues, Reforms.* Upper Saddle River, NJ: Prentice-Hall.

Light, Donald W. 2000a. "Sociological Perspectives on Competition in Health Care." *Journal of Health Politics, Policy and Law* 25(5): 969–974.

———. 2000b. "The Sociological Character of Health Care Markets." In *Handbook of Social Studies in Health and Medicine,* ed. Gary L. Albrecht, Ray Fitzpatrick, and Susan C. Scrimshaw. London: Sage.

Ludvigsen, Carol, and Kathleen Roberts. 1996. *Health Care Policies and Europe: The Implications for Practice.* Oxford: Butterworth-Heinemann.

Luft, Harold S. 1994. "Health Maintenance Organizations: Is the United States Experience Applicable Elsewhere?" In *Health: Quality and Choice.* Health Policy Studies No. 4. Organization for Economic Cooperation and Development. Paris, France.

Mackenbach, J.P. 1991. "Health Care Expenditure and Mortality from Amenable Conditions in the European Community." *Health Policy* 19: 245–255.

Matcha, Duane A. 2000. *Medical Sociology*. Boston: Allyn & Bacon.

———. (ed). 2001. *Readings in Medical Sociology*. Boston: Allyn & Bacon.

Matcha, Duane A., and Bonita A. Sessing-Matcha. 2001. "The Politics of Universal Health Care in the United States." Paper presented at the Medical Sociology Research Roundtables, American Sociological Association Meetings, Anaheim, CA, August.

McKeehan, Irina V. 1995. "Planning of National Primary Health Care and Prevention Programs: The First Health Insurance Law of Russia, 1991–1993." In *Global Perspectives on Health Care*, ed. Eugene B. Gallagher and Janardan Subedi. Englewood Cliffs, NJ: Prentice-Hall.

Mechanic, David, and David A. Rochefort. 1996. "Comparative Medical Systems." *Annual Review of Sociology* 22: 239–270.

Medical Expenditure Panel Survey. 2001. *"The Uninsured in America—1999."* Number 13. U.S. Department of Health and Human Services. Agency for Healthcare Research and Quality. Rockville, MD.

Mezentseva, Elena, and Natalia Rjmachevskaya. 1990. "The Soviet Country Profile: Health of the U.S.S.R. Population in the 70s and 80s—An Approach to a Comprehensive Analysis." *Social Science & Medicine* 31(8): 867–877.

Narine, Lutchmie. 2000. "Impact of Health Service Factors on Changes in Human Resource and Expenditures Levels in OECD Countries." *Journal of Health and Human Services Administration* 22(3): 292–307.

National Center for Health Statistics. 2000. *Health, United States, 2000*. Hyattsville, MD: Government Printing Office.

Navarro, Vicente. 1993. "Health Services Research: What Is It? A Review of *Health Services Research: An Anthology*, ed. K.L. White, J. Frenk, C. Ordonez, J.M. Paganini, and B. Starfield. Published by the Pan American Health Organization, 1992, *International Journal of Health Services* 23(1): 1–13.

Organization for Economic Cooperation and Development. 1994. *The Reform of Health Care Systems: A Review of Seventeen OECD Countries*. Paris, France.

———. 2000. *OECD Health Data 2000: A Comparative Analysis of 29 Countries*. Paris, France.

Orosz, Eva. 1990. "The Hungarian Country Profile: Inequalities in Health and Health Care in Hungary." *Social Science & Medicine* 31(8): 847–857.

Pfaff, Martin. 1990. "Differences in Health Care Spending across Countries: Statistical Evidence." *Journal of Health Politics, Policy and Law* 15(1): 1–67.

Raffel, Marshall W. 1997. "Dominant Issues: Convergence, Decentralization, Competition, Health Services." In *Health Care and Reform in Industrialized Countries*, ed. Marshall W. Raffel. University Park: Pennsylvania University Press.

Roemer, Milton I. 1991. *The Countries*. Vol. 1 of *National Health Systems of the World*. New York: Oxford.

———. 1994. "Recent Health System Development in Poland and Hungary." *Journal of Community Health* 19(3): 153–163.

Saltman, Richard B., and Joseph Figueras. 1997. *European Health Care Reform: Analysis of Current Strategies*. World Health Organization, WHO Regional Publications, European Series, No. 72. Regional Office for Europe. Copenhagen, Denmark.

————. 1998. "Analyzing the Evidence on European Health Care Reforms." *Health Affairs* 17(2): 85–108.

Scheil-Adlung, Xenia. 1998. "Steering the Healthcare Ship: Effects of Market Incentives to Control Costs in Selected OECD Countries." *International Social Security Review* 51(1): 103–136.

Schieber, George J., and Jean-Pierre Poullier. 1990. "Overview of International Comparisons of Health Care Expenditures." In *Health Care Systems in Transition: The Search for Efficiency.* Organization for Economic Cooperation and Development Social Policy Studies, No. 7. Paris, France.

Schoen, Cathy, Erin Strumpf, Karen Davis, Robin Osborn, Karen Donelan, and Robert J. Blendon. 2000. "The Elderly's Experiences with Health Care in Five Nations." New York: Commonwealth Fund.

Unschuld, Paul U. 1979. "Comparative Systems of Health Care." *Social Science & Medicine* 13A(5): 523–527.

U.S. Bureau of the Census. 2000. *Statistical Abstract of the United States: 2000,* 120th edition. Washington, DC: Government Printing Office.

van de Ven, Wynand P. M. M. 1996. "Market-Oriented Health Care Reforms: Trends and Future Options." *Social Science & Medicine* 43(5): 655–666.

Wessen, Albert F. 1999. "The Comparative Study of Health Care Reform." In *Health Care Systems in Transition: An International Perspective,* ed. Francis D. Powell and Albert F. Wessen. Thousand Oaks, CA: Sage.

White, Joseph. 1995. *Competing Solutions: American Health Care Proposals and International Solutions.* Washington, DC: Brookings Institution.

Whiteford, Linda M., and Lois Lacivita Nixon. 2000. "Comparative Health Systems: Emerging Convergences and Globalization." In *Handbook of Social Studies in Health and Medicine,* ed. Gary L. Albrecht, Ray Fitzpatrick, and Susan C. Scrimshaw. London: Sage.

Whitehead, Margaret. 1992. "The Concepts and Principles of Equity and Health." *International Journal of Health Services* 22(3): 429–445.

————. 1998. "Diffusion of Ideas on Social Inequalities in Health: A European Perspective." *Milbank Quarterly* 76(3): 469–492.

Wnuk-Lipinski, Edmund. 1990. "The Polish Country Profile: Economic Crisis and Inequalities in Health." *Social Science & Medicine* 31(8): 859–866.

World Health Organization. 1997. *Health in Europe 1997. Report on the Third Evaluation of Progress Towards Health for All in the European Region of WHO (1996–1997).* European Series, No. 83. Copenhagen: World Health Organization Regional Office for Europe.

————. 2000. *The World Health Report Health Systems: Improving Performance.* Geneva, Switzerland.

# Index

**About the Author**

DUANE A. MATCHA is Associate Professor of Sociology at Siena College in Loudonville, New York.